DIVINE
HEALING

A comprehensive guide
to nature's greatest
healing miracles

Fred Pescatore, M.D.

OV5B000557

Table of Contents

FOREWARD 1

PART I: Simple Natural Secrets to Life's Annoying Ailments:
The ultimate guide to everyday illness—from IBS to LDL

Chapter 1: A foolproof guide to a cold- & flu-proof immunity 5

Chapter 2: TBC: The Tree Bark CURE-ALL: How nature's
oldest and simplest material can save you from
sunburn, stroke...and everything in between 12

Chapter 3: Head-to-toe healing with Nature's
piece-of-cake cures 18

Chapter 4: The natural prescription for a PAIN-FREE life 54

Chapter 5: A simple sugar shot soothes pain in up to
90% of patients 79

Chapter 6: The silent enemy that's stealing your sleep...
and the drug-free prescription that will put your
insomnia to bed... 81

Chapter 7: 15 Foods that feed your sexual appetite—
no "little blue pill" required! 95

Chapter 8: The hidden "wine barrel secret" for curing
chronic fatigue...and much more 99

PART II: Shockingly Simple Cures for Today's Biggest Killers

Chapter 9: TauPro: The revolutionary sleep secret that
fights Alzheimer's too... 107

Chapter 10: The Halo Cure: A cut-poison-and-burn-free
solution for defying your diagnosis...................................... 111

Chapter 11: The "Mediterranean Miracle Molecule" that
strips cancer cells of their "superpower" and
kills them on sight 116

Chapter 12: The Complete Remission Blueprint:
Your personal guide to beating cancer with SP-5 120

Chapter 13: The Master Plan: How you can beat
cancer with curcumin 131

Chapter 14: Top Secret Triple-Threat Cure: How you can
wipe out the hidden epidemic of the baby
boomer generation 140

Chapter 15: Cholesterol's "Silent Partner": A statin-free
blueprint for avoiding heart attack and stroke...................... 148

Chapter 16: The 72-hour secret to a heart that's STRONG AS STEEL! 155

Chapter 17: Natural secrets to reverse Alzheimer's
disease and strengthen your brain 171

Chapter 18: 1 Hour Memory Breakthrough! Squash "senior
moments" with the Bavarian Brain Booster.............................187

**PART III: The New Hamptons Health Miracle: The next generation cure
for diabetes, pre-diabetes, belly fat, metabolic syndrome,
and so much more**

Chapter 19: 10 Diabetes Myths That Could Kill You 193

Chapter 20: Diabetes-Free in Just 6 Weeks...204

Chapter 21: Diabetes Cheat Sheet for Even Faster Results:
Without eating less or lifting a finger 219

Chapter 22: The Decadent Dining Out Plan: How to eat out
every day, still lose weight, AND defeat diabetes 234

Chapter 23: Amazing Hamburger Cure: How to cure
obesity for life, with the help of America's
favorite "junk food" 243

Chapter 24: The 3-Day Sugar Cure: Start reversing
diabetes in just 72 hours.. 246

Chapter 25: The Top Secret Super Charger—One secret
ingredient that makes dodging diabetes simple.................. 253

PART IV: Decadent Diet-Free Recipes

Chapter 26: BREAKFAST: Never be bored again 260

Chapter 27: LUNCH: Enjoy all these "forbidden" favorites.................... 272

Chapter 28: DINNERS: Dine in decadence! 284

Chapter 27: SAVORY SIDES 302

Chapter 30: Sweet and Sinful Desserts... 306

SOURCES 315

FOREWARD

Twenty-five years ago I witnessed the many failures of modern American medicine on the frontlines as an ER doctor in New York. After just 6 months of watching the same sick patients sent home with the same failed treatments time after time… I had seen enough. Since then I've learned to combine the best of both modern and natural medicine in such far off places as Asia, India, Japan, Africa and Europe. And while I've watched these techniques work modern day miracles for my patients over the last two decades, American medicine seems to have only gotten worse and worse.

Billions have been gutted from life-saving medical research programs, almost 20 percent of critical medical scientists are considering leaving the country, and doctors are turning away Medicare patients by the tens of thousands. Put simply, American medicine is on life support.

Big Pharma would like you to believe prescription drugs are the only way out. 92 percent of seniors have at least one chronic condition, and take an average of 20 prescriptions per year. But the facts are the facts: This country is not getting any healthier. And that's why I've decided to release this guide to drug-free healing, filled with some of the most powerful natural alternative secrets known to medicine. Big Pharma may deny the existence of these cures, but I've seen the proof that it works in my own patients.

In the following pages, I'll provide you with the tools you need to heal and protect yourself during these frightening times of medical uncertainty.

To health and longevity for years to come,

Fred Pescatore, M.D.
Editor, *Logical Health Alternatives*

PART 1

SIMPLE NATURAL SECRETS TO LIFE'S ANNOYING AILMENTS

The ultimate guide to everyday illness—from IBS to LDL

Chapter 1

A foolproof guide to a
cold- & flu-proof immunity

It's a fact, every second of every day your immune system is under constant attack.

But there's one immune-destroying compound in particular that's growing to epidemic proportions throughout the world. In fact, The World Health Organization considers it one of the top 10 most dangerous chemicals to your health.

But unlike other chemicals and compounds on that list, this one is so common it's almost impossible to avoid completely. I'm talking about mercury. And if you were living almost anywhere but the U.S. you'd already be taking measures to limit your exposure.

In fact, in October of 2013 an international convention was held in Japan where ...

Over 90 countries signed a global treaty
to cut their citizens' exposure to this immune-killing
chemical...But guess who's not on the list!

You guessed it, the good old U.S. government.

It was called the Minamata Convention and virtually every industrialized country you can think of recognized the growing danger mercury poses to its citizens: Canada, the UK, Germany, France, Japan... Heck even China—where pollution standards are so low the surgical-mask has become a fashion staple—signed this treaty!

Meanwhile, you're still more exposed than ever. And the danger is right in your own home!

In fact, in September 2013, the WHO sent out an urgent warning to avoid these 7 common household items that increase your exposure to mercury:

- batteries
- measuring devices, such as thermometers and barometers
- electric switches and relays in equipment
- lamps (including some types of light bulbs)
- dental amalgam (for dental fillings)
- skin-lightening products and other cosmetics
- pharmaceuticals

Mercury is also found in foods, especially fish.

Obviously, I'm not telling you to stop eating fish. That would be ridiculous. But you must be choosy about the types of seafood you eat.

Large predators—like swordfish, tilefish, tuna, and shark—are loaded with mercury. Do yourself a favor and avoid them.

Lower mercury options include catfish, herring, pollock, haddock, tilapia, and wild-caught salmon. Generally speaking, you can eat as many as three servings of these fish per week.

And of course, if you take fish oil (and I absolutely recommend you do), be sure to select a safe, purified supplement to get your fill of omega-3s. (Though more often than not, fish oil is derived from small fish like anchovies and sardines, which are both naturally low in mercury anyway.)

The dangers of excessive mercury exposure really couldn't get any clearer

But unfortunately, it's a condition that easily falls through the cracks, with symptoms that mimic a long list of other common diseases. (We're talking everything from memory loss and depression to joint pain, fatigue, and allergies.)

That's one reason why I routinely test my patients for mercury toxicity. And believe me, positive results are not at all uncommon.

So by all means, I recommend having your own mercury levels tested if you're displaying any of the above symptoms

Unfortunately, it's nearly impossible to avoid mercury completely. It's in the air we breathe, the food we eat and the water we drink... Which is a big part of why this is becoming such a problem! So what else can you do?

The immune-boosting powerhouse that takes on all concerns

One ingredient I've been recommending for years is a veritable jack-of-all-trades immunity breakthrough known as beta-glucans.

Beta-glucans are sugars found in the cell walls of bacteria, fungi and plants such as oats and barley. They already have a reputation as an immune-boosting powerhouse used by people whose body defenses have been weakened by conditions such as chronic fatigue syndrome, or physical and emotional stress; or by treatments such as radiation or chemotherapy.

Beta-glucans are also used for the common cold, flu, H1N1 (swine) flu, allergies, hepatitis, Lyme disease, asthma, ear infections, aging, ulcerative colitis and Crohn's disease, fibromyalgia, rheumatoid arthritis, and multiple sclerosis.

And it's one of the only natural substances I know of powerful enough to fight the immune-damaging effects of mercury exposure head-on.

With this level of immune supporting power you might expect to pay a pretty penny for beta-glucans but you can actually get them for as little as 33 pennies a day! Beta-glucans are readily available online with some 30 day supplies going for as little as $9.99.

But be certain to check the amount of beta-glucans you're getting in every dose. I usually recommend a dosage of at least 70 mg a day for optimal protection.

Beta-glucans are one of the most powerful immune-supporting ingredients around but if preliminary studies on this next compound hold up, it could make beta-glucans look like Tic-Tacs!

It all started over 20 years ago when one researcher set out to answer a question that's stumped scientists for decades...

Why are sharks completely immune to all known viruses?

It's a mystery that's kept sharks at the top of the food chain for hundreds of millions of years...

And when Dr. Michael Zasloff of Georgetown University studied the shark's remarkable immune system...he found the key.

It's an extraordinary "golden particle" compound known as squalamine and according to Dr. Zasloff, it's...

"Like nothing else that has ever been described or discovered."

Why? Because unlike vaccines, which need to be specifically tailored to each and every individual virus, squalamine works by exploiting a weakness shared by every virus known to man—the need to feed.

From the common cold to HIV, when a virus enters your cells, the first thing it does is feast on positively charged proteins in your cell walls in order to replicate and spread.

But when the squalamine enters a cell, it pops these proteins off without harming the cell... Leaving nothing behind for the virus to feed on!

And again, according to Dr. Zasloff...

"There is no other compound known to science that does this—this is a remarkable property."

And to prove it, squalamine was lab-tested on some of the most deadly viruses known to man...

And to everyone's surprise, this "golden particle" not only prevented, but killed viruses such as dengue fever, yellow fever, and hepatitis A and D (just to name a few)!

You read that right…Lab tests show the squalamine can prevent and kill viruses that currently have no known vaccine!

In fact, squalamine can effectively defend against and eradicate over 194 different viruses in the lab... And fast! Studies show the squalamine can go to work in just hours.

So why hasn't squalamine gotten more mainstream attention? Because like with most natural breakthroughs, instead of being presented in its natural form, pharmaceutical companies are rushing to create a synthesized version so they can cash in!

But you can get the same natural version of squalamine that showed so much promise in lab tests right this moment!

Squalamine is generally found in shark liver oil which is readily available online. Shark liver oil supplements are available through a number of major manufacturers—Life Extension, Country Life, and Puritan's Pride, to name a few. I generally recommend a dose of 1,000 mg, twice per day to raise white blood cell counts—a benefit that will strengthen your body's defenses against everything— from cancer to the common cold.

Flu-proof your immune system in just three days

Come every Fall, the flu shot propaganda is in full swing. So I always take the time to remind readers that the flu vaccine isn't all it's cracked up to be. I never, ever get a flu shot. And guess what? I never get sick, either. Because I follow my own common-sense advice when it comes to staying healthy during cold and flu season.

That advice goes like this:

- Eliminate sugar

- Wash your hands regularly (with plain, old soap and water— NOT anti-bacterial soaps and gels)

- Take 1,000 mg of AHCC per day

This protocol offers just as much protection as the flu shot (if not more)…with a whole lot less risk.

Yes, warding off colds and the flu really is THAT simple.

But I recently came across some new research that points to an intriguing addition to this basic flu-prevention strategy. (And it *still* doesn't require a shot.)

Get this: Researchers think that fasting—that's right, *fasting*—may be the secret to regenerating a weakened immune system.

Recent studies show that undergoing several two- to four-day fasting cycles, staggered over the course of six months can flip a switch that puts your immune system into "turnover" mode.

That's because, when you're fasting, your body attempts to conserve energy by cutting the fat—literally and figuratively. It burns through fat and sugar stores for energy, while culling worn out white blood cells that aren't pulling their weight anymore.

At the same time, your levels of an enzyme called PKA start to lower. And this eventually sends signals to your body to start producing new, healthy immune cells. (It's worth mentioning that prolonged fasting also lowers levels of IGF-1—the same hormone implicated in tumor growth.)

The end result is a rehabbed immune system. And you don't even have to lift a finger.

This strategy could have some pretty amazing applications. In fact, this team of scientists found that prolonged fasting reduced levels of circulating PKA—and put the brakes on chemotherapy-related immunosuppression and mortality—in mice.

Which would mean nothing, of course, if the results didn't happen to coincide with the outcome of a previous pilot study. That Phase I clinical trial showed that prolonged fasting in *humans*—in this case, during the 72 hours prior to chemotherapy—can protect white blood cells and ward off toxicity as well.

So just *imagine* what it might do for someone who's simply trying to avoid the flu. Fasting may also prove to be a real game-changer when it comes to immunosenesence—or, as I call it, immunity rot.

This condition is the gradual breakdown of immunity that results from aging…and it has potentially deadly consequences. If these new results hold water, fasting could play a key role in stopping this silent epidemic in its tracks.

Obviously, this is still very new research. But it's not the first time science has uncovered impressive benefits simply from fasting. (And not just as a weight-loss strategy—fasting can curb high blood sugar, lower cholesterol and blood pressure, and cut inflammation, too.)

So whether or not this tactic can spare you from the latest bug making the rounds, I'm still a big proponent of responsible, properly planned fasting. Nothing drastic—just 24 to 48 hours, with plenty of water.

I do this once a month myself, and I always feel refreshed and energized afterwards.

Chapter 2

TBC: The Amazing
Tree Bark CURE-ALL

How Nature's oldest and simplest material can save you from sunburn, stroke... and everything in between

In all my years dedicated to overturning the mainstream medical dogma and developing the simplest—most effective—healing cures, I've never come across one quite as PERFECT as this.

There's simply no easier way to make such an enormous impact on every aspect of your health. From the top of your head to the tip of your toe.

Even deadly serious conditions like Alzheimer's and hypertension are no match for this natural remedy. And you'd *never guess* the source...

This virtual cure-all comes from one of nature's oldest, simplest materials...

Tree bark, of all things!

But before you start chipping away at the old maple in your backyard, hang on just a second!

I'm not talking about any old tree bark here. No, this one is highly unique.

It comes from a particular type of pine tree that only grows along the southwest coast of France, in the Les Landes de Gascogne area. And inside this exotic pine bark is an extract called Pycnogenol.®

Since researchers began looking at it more closely over 60 years ago, more than 220 studies have been published on the benefits of Pycnogenol—demonstrating its antioxidant properties, its ability to help reduce blood sugar, its effects on cardiovascular and circulatory health, and much, MUCH more.

From the outside in and back again, this remarkable extract works wonders for what ails you…

Nature's own ALLERGY medicine

Silence those hay fever symptoms without the brain fog or heavy head! Allergy meds work by keeping sneeze-triggering histamine from attaching to your cells.

But this little wonder does Allegra one better.

Pycnogenol can help prevent the release of histamine in the first place, keeping you allergy-free from the start.

Erase the NO. 2 FEAR of getting older

Cancer reigns supreme as the biggest fear of getting older. But close on cancer's heels, is something many of us take for granted until it's too late—vision loss.

But Pycnogenol has been shown to sharpen vision like Windex on a dirty window. Plus, it halts the primary cause of cataracts—free-radical damage—stopping it in its tracks. And helps defend against retinopathy.

Forget the "LITTLE BLUE PILL"

Get back the stamina and performance you had in your 20s. Yep! Pycnogenol is a miracle worker for erectile dysfunction. In fact, it operates in a similar way to Viagra…but naturally. (In other words—without the risk!)

You see, Pycnogenol helps keep your blood vessels healthy, so blood and oxygen can flow freely to every area of your body. And blood and oxygen are two critical elements in achieving and maintaining an erection.

So is another substance called nitric oxide (NO). And Pycnogenol helps boost your body's natural NO production.

Best of all…combining Pycnogenol and another NO-booster known as

L-arginine could mean twice as much sex. In a study involving patients with mild to moderate erectile dysfunction, 92.5% of men responded well to this combination. The study dose was 40 mg of Pycnogenol and 1.5 g of L-arginine aspartate, taken twice a day for four weeks.

But this nutrient is not just for men...

Relieve the 6 most dreaded symptoms of menopause

A group of Italian researchers enrolled 70 women in their study. Thirty-eight took 100 mg Pycnogenol daily for an 8-week period, and 32 women did not. Researchers evaluated 33 common signs and symptoms of menopause before the study's start, and at its end.

Six of the most common symptoms—hot flashes, night sweats, mood swings, irregular periods, loss of libido, and vaginal dryness—were decreased in the Pycnogenol group. The control group had no changes.

The Pycnogenol group also showed relief from fatigue, sleeping disorders, concentration and memory problems, dizziness, depression and irritability. Although those findings did not show up as "statistically significant."

The researchers measured damaging "oxidative stress" in the women by measuring free radicals in the small blood vessels. Oxidative stress was significantly lowered after four and eight weeks. No changes in the control group.

Hush that incessant RINGING in your ears

Hissing, ringing, buzzing. Day in and day out. If you've got tinnitus, you know just how maddening it can be. Even worse—most doctors will tell you there's "nothing you can do."

But I've been tracking the research on Pycnogenol for close to a decade now. And just a few years ago, a group of Italian researchers put it to the test in 82 tinnitus patients. And just 150 milligrams of Pycnogenol reduced tinnitus symptoms by more than 62%.

It's a small study—and not a fool-proof cure. But if you suffer with tinnitus, you know ANY dent in your symptoms is a miracle!

Armor your brain against ALZHEIMER'S disease

Research on Pycnogenol for Alzheimer's is just taking off, and already it's showing some amazing results.

It helps stop the No. 1 marker of Alzheimer's—dangerous beta-amyloid plaque—from killing off brain cells. And one randomized trial showed Pycnogenol improved memory and everyday thinking in elderly patients.

Shield yourself from SUNBURN—
from the inside out

I know it sounds crazy, but with Pycnogenol you can shield yourself from dangerous UV rays—with a SIMPLE PILL.

In one study, researchers found that when volunteers supplemented with Pycnogenol for four weeks, they didn't sunburn as easily following exposure to UV light.

In other words, Pycnogenol can actually give you a built-in SPF, without the dangerous chemicals in lotions, oils, and sprays.

The safest STROKE prevention on the planet

Think of it like Nature's Coumadin…keeping your blood clot-free and flowing with ease. But much, much safer than prescription blood thinners—or even aspirin!

(And if you love to travel—don't forget the Pycnogenol in your carry-on: It works for deep vein thrombosis and swelling, too.)

And that's just the beginning of what
Pycnogenol can do for you!

Just look at what else Pycnogenol is capable of. It also…

- Shaves <u>days</u> off of wound-healing time—and prevents ugly, disfiguring scars

- Promotes a youthful, glowing, *wrinkle-free* complexion

- Sooths the itching, scaly skin of psoriasis

- Even helps kids with ADHD—one study showed that within a month, symptoms were barely noticeable!

Plus, this remarkable tree bark cure even plays a major role in curbing impaired microcirculation—the culprit behind so many of today's biggest health threats. In fact it's one of the primary components of my "Triple Threat Cure" in Chapter 12.

Clinical research has shown that one of the primary ways Pycnogenol benefits your microcirculation is by targeting collagen and elastin, which are the building blocks that line your blood vessels.

Unfortunately, a combination of aging and less-than-ideal food choices cause collagen and elastin to break down. But Pycnogenol helps the body replenish these two critical substances—and keeps your blood vessels working the way they're supposed to in the process.

Recommended dosages

As you can see, there's almost nothing Pycnogenol can't do. Which is why I recommend it to all of my patients. Dosage can vary depending on the nature of any specific health concern. Minimum dosage for general antioxidant protection is 20 mg. For general health, I recommend 50 to 100 mg per day.

Higher doses of 100 mg per day can be taken for heart-health concerns, such as high blood pressure, blood clotting, and impaired circulation.

If you have diabetes or blood sugar concerns, you may need additional support. I have my diabetes patients take 100 to 200 mg of Pycnogenol per day.

For osteoarthritis or asthma, 100 mg per day is recommended.

Pycnogenol may cause some gastrointestinal discomfort. This can be due to the astringent nature of the extract. Taking it with or after meals may help reduce any GI symptoms.

Pycnogenol supplements (and supplement formulas that contain it) are actually widely available in many vitamin shops and even in natural food stores. They can be on the pricey side. But when you consider all the potential benefits this one, single extract has to offer—it's actually one of the best investments you can make in your health.

One note of caution—Pycnogenol is actually a patented extract, so make sure any product you choose lists it with the registered trademark symbol (Pycnogenol®). Otherwise, it may not be the real deal—or provide the same benefits.

Chapter 3

Head-to-toe healing with Nature's piece-of-cake cures

One food everyone with allergies should avoid

You can't escape it. In fall, the air is full of pollen from ragweed and mold spores that grow in damp leaf piles. In spring, budding trees and flowers release their own pollen. And in the winter, simply turning on the furnace churns up dust mites. These factors alone are enough to make you miserable, if you've got allergies. But there are some things that might be contributing to your symptoms that you CAN control—and some of them might surprise you...

If you're sensitive to ragweed and mold, for instance, you might be eating things that can cause similar sniffling, sneezing, and itchiness.

You see, certain foods are genetically related "cousins" to allergens like ragweed, grasses, or trees. And I'm not talking about genetic modifications here. These plants are simply in the same species, so your body can have a similar sort of reaction to them. For example:

- **If you're sensitive to ragweed**, your immune system may react to foods like corn, tomatoes, melon, apples, peaches, pears, apricots, cherries, berries, plums, bananas, cucumbers, squash, or chamomile tea.

- **During spring allergy season**, when trees and grasses release their pollen, foods like apple, pear, kiwi, cherry, parsley, peach, carrots, and even some nuts (almonds or walnuts) can trigger an allergic reaction.

- **If you're allergic to mold**—which is a common allergen in fall and winter, in leaves and in damp, dark spaces like basements—it's best to avoid foods that have been fermented or contain mold, fungi, or yeast—like cheese, sour cream, mushrooms, beer or wine, and vinegar-based foods like salad dressings.

Keep in mind, not everyone has this type of cross-reaction with foods... but if you're battling a seasonal allergy, think about the foods you're eating, and try cutting back on or eliminating the foods listed above to see if it makes a difference for you. And don't forget about **the one food <u>everyone</u> with allergies should avoid.**

I'm talking, of course, about SUGAR.

Sugar is a major threat to your immune system. In fact, even <u>one teaspoon of sugar can suppress the immune system by 56 percent!</u> And a compromised immune system is even less likely to be able to handle allergens. Unfortunately, you might be taking in more sugar than you realize.

Simple carbs like white bread, crackers, and pastries are obvious sources. But a glass of orange juice contains two teaspoons (or more) sugar. And even certain fruits—like apples, kiwis, and oranges—are especially high in sugar. When you cut these from your everyday diet, you'll give your gut health (and your immune system) a big boost, and you'll be another step forward in curbing allergies.

The misunderstood nutrient you need to eat more of

Protein is a key component in weight management, metabolism, healthy aging, and an overall healthy diet. Yet conventional doctors and nutrition "experts" can't agree on how much protein we need for optimum health. (Hint: Their recommendations are much too low based on the prevailing research.)

But the good news is, this is slowly changing, thanks in part to a pair of international Protein Summits held during the last decade. Their goal was to discuss the role of protein in human health and to explore the misperception that Americans eat too much of it. These summits finally reinforced what we already knew: that a higher protein intake contributes to better nutrition, healthy weight management, and more lean body mass.

Finally, protein is taking its rightful place at the head of the table—the breakfast, lunch, and dinner table, that is. So how much protein do you really need?

New science calls for more protein

Based on the government's current Recommended Daily Allowance (RDA), a 150-pound person should consume just 54 grams of protein per day. But nearly all of the recent research on protein indicates this amount is far too low.

After taking the new research into account, I recommend 1 gram of protein per pound you weigh. And if you're trying to gain weight or build muscle, I often recommend twice that amount.

Why so much? After all, my recommendation is almost triple the RDA (or as I like to call it, the Ridiculous Daily Allowance). Well, study after study backs me up.

Protein and weight loss. An overview of studies on protein's role in weight management addresses key topics like protein's influence on satiety, and how even small changes in protein intake can increase your body's energy expenditure. In plain English, that means it can help keep you fuller for longer, as well as rev up your metabolism and help you burn more calories. Which, of course, helps you lose weight.

The researchers found that weight-loss diets focused on higher protein consumption (about 0.5 to 0.75 grams for every pound of body weight) led to modest weight loss in less than three months.

"Modest" weight loss doesn't seem very exciting. But the researchers point out that small changes in weight are often underappreciated, even though they are beneficial to our health. Just like with blood pressure—a little improvement goes a long way.

Protein and muscle mass. Another new study shows that daily protein intake of at least 0.5 grams per pound of body weight can help improve muscle mass, strength, and function in older adults.

So to preserve your muscle mass and strength as you age, you need to boost your protein consumption.

The researchers also note that in addition to total protein, the amount of protein you eat at each meal also has an effect on your muscles. They conclude that older adults should eat a minimum of 30 grams of protein per meal.

Because physical activity enhances muscle protein synthesis, the researchers also suggest that protein recommendations be linked to how much a person exercises. Again, this isn't really news to me—or to you. But it still encourages me that protein and all its benefits are taking the main stage now.

A quick—and tasty— way to boost your protein intake

By all means you should start by including protein in every meal. And don't forget, protein doesn't always have to come in the form of meat. Eggs, cheese, and nuts are all great sources of protein.

Ask Dr. Fred
An allergen-free protein boost

Q: "You suggest using whey protein to prevent losing muscle. But I'm allergic to casein and whey. Can I use your WheyLogic or something comparable without having a major reaction?"

A: If you were only casein sensitive, then WheyLogic would be a great choice. But since you are also allergic to whey, I recommend you look at products that use organic pea protein or hemp protein instead.

I also recommend taking a good probiotic as well as a GI-support supplement. Enter "digestive support" in the search box at www.drpesca-tore.com to learn more. Your body will thank you in the end.

But you may find you still need more. After all, 1 gram per pound of body weight is a lot of protein. Especially when you consider that a 4-ounce serving of steak only contains 28 grams of protein. And a three-egg veggie omelet packs a petite 18 grams.

That's why I recommend at least one whey protein shake a day. Whey protein is an easy—and tasty—way to add 20 or more grams of protein to your daily total. (For instance, a single scoop of my WheyLogic contains a whopping 21 grams of protein.)

Just remember there are a few things to consider when choosing a whey protein product. Look for one that has 8 grams of carbs or less per serving. And mix it with plain water. If you like a thicker consistency, add some ice cubes and mix it up in a blender. You can add a tablespoon of macadamia nut oil for a healthy boost of monounsaturated fatty acids (this little trick will also keep you full even longer).

Warning: "Gluten free" doesn't mean allergen free

Many of my patients seem to believe all gluten-free foods are created equal. I've said it before, but I'll say it again: Just because something's gluten-free, doesn't mean it's good for you. Especially if it's a pre-packaged, processed "food" loaded with preservatives. And now there's even more reason to stay away from these junk foods in disguise.

Apparently, a number of gluten-free products here in the U.S. are starting to include a legume called lupin, which is used frequently in other countries. This yellow-colored bean is particularly popular in Europe, Mediterranean countries, Australia and New Zealand.

Here's what's so concerning: Lupin contains the same protein that causes allergic reactions to peanuts and soybeans. But since it's not a nut, people who have peanut or soy allergies don't know to look for it on labels. Obviously, this can be very dangerous—downright deadly, even.

But despite the risks, lupin is expected to become more popular because it's high in protein and fiber and low in fat. (A perfect trifecta for food manufacturers, and their advertising teams.)

Supposedly, the FDA is "actively monitoring complaints of lupin allergies by U.S. consumers." But I won't hold my breath for them to do anything about it anytime soon.

If you've got a peanut, soy, or other legume allergy, make sure to look for lupin on the label of ANY food you pick up in the supermarket. But, once again, your best bet is to skip packaged, processed foods altogether—"gluten-free" or otherwise.

The #1 disease-fighting green vegetable

You may have only heard of **watercress** as an ingredient in sandwiches served with fancy English teas. But this leafy green is much more than that. In fact, it's so nutritious that I call it the "new kale."

Like kale, watercress is loaded with vitamins, minerals, antioxidants, and other nutrients. But watercress has even more of a nutritional punch than kale. According to a recent study from the Centers for Disease Control (CDC) rating "powerhouse" produce, watercress has a perfect 100-nutrient density score.

That makes it No. 1 among the CDC's 41 fruits and vegetables most likely to reduce your risk of chronic disease.

Think about that…Watercress has more nutrient density than chard (number three on the list) or spinach (number five). Where does kale rank? All the way down at number 15!

The irony is that watercress hardly looks like a plant stuffed with nutrients. Its leaves and stems are small and delicate. And it's picky about where it grows. It likes water, so you'll find it near springs and waterways, or cultivated in hydroponic greenhouses.

Watercress has a slightly bitter, peppery taste like arugula, mustard greens, and cress—its botanical cousins. It's a great addition to salads, soups, or even

Watercress Scramble with Garlic

Yield: 1 serving

INGREDIENTS

1 teaspoon macadamia nut oil

1 clove garlic, minced

1 cup watercress (stems removed or diced if you prefer)

2 large eggs

Coarse salt and freshly ground black pepper

DIRECTIONS

Heat oil in a small skillet over medium heat. Add garlic and cook until fragrant, about 1 minute. Add watercress and cook, stirring, until just wilted. Remove from pan and set aside. Lower heat to medium-low.

Whisk eggs and season with salt and pepper. Pour eggs into pan and cook, stirring, until just set. Return watercress to pan and stir.

as a topper on grilled steak.

Cancer prevention. Research shows a compound in watercress can significantly reduce one of the most important cancer triggers—DNA damage in cells. And it can also help your cells resist DNA damage in the future. The study participants ate 2 ½ cups of watercress a day for eight weeks. You can easily toss the same amount in your daily salad and still have room for plenty of other healthy greens and veggies.

Another study of breast cancer survivors found that just a single serving of watercress may turn off a signal in the body that feeds tumors. So the more watercress you eat, the more you starve cancerous tumors.

Building strong bones and fighting osteoporosis. Watercress is loaded with vitamin K, calcium, and manganese—all key bone-building nutrients.

Eye health. Watercress is rich in vitamin A, lutein, and zeaxanthin, which help prevent age-related eye issues like macular degeneration.

Immunity. Along with vitamin A, watercress is also a good source of vitamin C. Both of these nutrients help keep our immune systems functioning at their best. And that means fewer colds, not to mention less risk of more serious diseases.

Considering all that watercress can do for your health, it's no surprise that ancient healers made sure to keep a supply of this leafy green handy. In fact, it's been said that Hippocrates himself built a hospital next to a stream so he could harvest fresh watercress any time a patient needed it.

You don't have to be that dedicated to get your daily health fix. You can find watercress in most natural foods stores, high-end groceries, or even Asian markets. And because it's often grown hydroponically in greenhouses, it's usually available year round.

Drop 7 points from your blood pressure in just 8 weeks

A number of studies show blueberries can significantly decrease blood pressure. In one study of postmenopausal women, just eight weeks of blueberry consumption lowered their blood pressure from 138/80 to 131/75.

And that was with no other lifestyle changes. So imagine if you threw in an extra hour of exercise with your weekly blueberry consumption. Or did something as simple as cutting white bread out of your diet. Chances are your blood pressure would drop even lower. Another study showed blueberries can also help reduce fat accumulation in white blood cells—which helps prevent the hardening of the arteries that leads to cardiovascular disease.

How to reap the benefits of berries even in the dead of winter

What do you do when organic berries are not in season?

I recommend getting your daily dose of berries in powder form. Superfood "purples" blends typically contain blueberries, blackberries and black raspberries—often along with other nutritional powerhouses like acai, figs, eggplant, beets, and purple carrots.

Add a scoop of a purples blend to a glass of water to create a tasty juice-like drink—but without all of the sugar and calories found in fruit juices. Or add it to a whey protein shake. You'll get the same health benefits you get from whole blueberries, blackberries, or black raspberries—no matter what season it is.

The blood-pressure remedy so easy you can do it in your sleep

Believe it or not, lack of quality sleep may be an important—and neglected—contributing factor in cases of hypertension.

Researchers at Harvard Medical School found that men who spent less than 4 percent of their sleep in "slow-wave sleep" were 83 percent more likely to develop high blood pressure by the study's end. These men had poorer-quality sleep—less hours of sleep, more awakenings, and more sleep apnea.

This is the first study to find that poor-quality sleep—not just lack of sleep—affects blood pressure.

If you're not getting 6-8 hours of restorative sleep each night, and you've already tried addressing the obvious culprits (cutting back on caffeine, establishing a relaxing bedtime routine, etc.), try taking a closer look at your actual surroundings.

It may not seem important (after all, you're asleep, right?) But the fact is, certain environmental factors can negatively affect how well you're sleeping.

One of the things I always recommend to my patients is to make sure they're sleeping in absolute darkness—even the light from the alarm clock can alter your sleep patterns. Also, try turning your thermostat down a few degrees before you turn in for the night. During the day, you're probably comfortable with a room temperature in the 70s, but studies show that an optimal sleeping temperature is between 60-68 degrees Farenheit.

And, above all, make sure that you're making sleep a priority. Your health depends on it.

The 20-minute outdoor trick that's curing high blood pressure

A new study out of University College London showed higher levels of vitamin D directly contribute to lower risk of hypertension and heart disease. Researchers looked at data from 35 studies and over 155,000 subjects. They also employed a special approach known as "Mendelian randomization." This method looks at genes in order to examine causality as opposed to correlation.

Up until now, most studies on vitamin D and heart health have only established links between the two.

This is among the first to establish a clear cause-and-effect relationship. Results showed that people with high concentrations of the sunshine vitamin had lower blood pressure overall. In fact, for every 10 percent increase in vitamin D concentrations, there was an 8.1 percent decrease in hypertension risk.

Now this is great news if you happen to live in an area with a warmer climate, where presumably everyone's getting a lot more sun. But if you've been hiding indoors, now's the time to get outside. All you need to boost your stores of vitamin D is 20 to 30 minutes of maximum exposure to mid-day sun.

It's the easiest half hour you might have all day. But if you live in a colder climate like I do, make sure you're taking a good supplement. I always recommend at least 2,000 IUs of vitamin D3 daily.

The secret prostate cure that's been hiding on your Thanksgiving dinner table for generations

You hear about women battling urinary tract infections all the time. But few doctors ever talk about treating men's urinary problems.

Their sole focus is on shrinking the prostate. And, don't get me wrong—that is important. But there's more to male "mechanics" than the prostate. The urethra has problems of its own, including inflammation that makes urinating very painful. And these issues are generally lumped together under one catch-all diagnosis: prostatitis.

Unfortunately, the catch-all treatment—antibiotics—is notoriously ineffective. In fact, there's not a single documented case that antibiotics are effective for treating the problems associated with prostatitis (like a burning sensation while urinating, pain in the perineum, blood in the urine, and painful ejaculation).

That's why for the past 15 years, I've been suggesting that my male patients use the same natural treatment women have been relying on to cure UTIs for generations: cranberry juice.

I admit, I didn't have a whole lot to go on the first time I recommended this approach. But it just made sense—if cranberry juice helps to keep the female urinary tract healthy, it should work for men, too. And it did. So I've continued prescribing it ever since. In fact, I have patient after patient who could tell you just how well cranberries work for guys. Take Ron, for example.

Here's what he has to say about cranberry:

"I'm 67 years old and have suffered a long time with having to urinate constantly throughout the day. It got so bad, I even kept a log and the worst day was 23 times. I went to a conventional urologist who tried me on all the usual drugs. They helped a little, but I didn't like the way they made me feel. And besides, I always preferred the more holistic approach. I was taking all of the nutritional supplements that I had read about for prostate health--saw palmetto, etc. But when I saw Dr. Fred, he mentioned starting cranberry. He said he had used it in many men who had no or little success with all the traditional supplements. So, I figured why not? Within 2 weeks I began to see an improvement--and within 8 weeks, I stopped keeping my log as I was down to about 6 trips to the bathroom per day, which, for me, was a fantastic improvement."

Now—finally—there's a study that backs me up in recommending cranberry to men like Ron.

Researchers in the Czech Republic have discovered the first firm evidence that cranberries may improve lower urinary tract symptoms in men.

The study, published in the *British Journal of Nutrition*, involved 42 men diagnosed with chronic non-bacterial prostatitis. Half the men took 1,500 mg of dried powdered cranberries daily for 6 months, while the control group took no cranberry treatment. Their prostate-related symptoms were taken at baseline, and at three and six months later.

Men who took the cranberry treatment had significant improvements in quality of life, urine flow and volume (and other factors measured by the International Prostate Symptom Score); and in levels of prostate-specific antigens, or PSA.

In other words, they could pee again easily—without the pain!

And other research is pointing to the potential for cranberry supplements to **prevent** repeated UTIs in women. (And my guess is it will do the same for men. Again, it just makes sense!)

This is very good news, especially since drinking too much cranberry juice might increase risk of kidney stones. Not to mention the fact that fruit juice is a notoriously overlooked contributor to sugar-overload, obesity, and diabetes.

Two new tests that could save your prostate—and your life

I still believe strongly in the PSA test. That said, there's no denying that this screening tool has contributed to the overdiagnosis and overtreatment problems running rampant in mainstream medicine today.

Consequently, millions of men have had their prostates butchered, based on a test that offers valuable but limited information. And they're now irreversibly incontinent and/or impotent because of it.

But like I've also said before, doing away with the PSA test isn't the answer here. Because it's not the PSA test's fault that these men had unnecessary surgery to treat a cancer that wouldn't likely have killed them anyway. The blame here lies with overzealous doctors making dubious treatment decisions.

The simple fact is, most cases of prostate cancer don't require any action unless the benefits outweigh the risks. And that circumstance only applies to the most aggressive, lethal forms of the disease.

And how do you know if your prostate cancer is the aggressive variety? Well, a major breakthrough in testing just made it a whole lot easier.

1. Prostate Health Index

This new blood test, called the Prostate Health Index (PHI), is based on prostate-specific antigen (PSA). But it factors in several different measurements—including total PSA, proenzyme PSA, and free PSA—to generate a single score that provides a more complete picture than any one individual measure.

Basically, if your free PSA is lower while the other forms of PSA are elevated, then you are more likely to have "clinically significant"—i.e., aggressive and potentially deadly—prostate cancer.

According to a number of different studies, this method of testing offers greater specificity than a single PSA test alone. It outperforms "regular" PSA testing when it comes to predicting high-grade prostate cancer. And it can also predict the likelihood that your cancer will progress. Both of which dramatically reduce the risk of unnecessary procedures in cases of low-risk disease.

So here's the bottom line: If your PSA is between 2 and 10 and you're wondering what to do, ask your doctor about this new testing.

I know you probably hate statistics, but this is an important one: Roughly 1.6 million American men get an annual blood test to assess for prostate cancer. Of these men, about 1 million will go on to get a biopsy. Out of that group, 750,000 men test negative.

Unfortunately, false negatives are common—so repeat biopsies are often carried out. But biopsies are invasive and painful. Not to mention the fact that aggravating cancer cells in this way can potentially cause them to spread.

But now there's a new, less invasive way to get the same information you could get from repeat biopsies...

2. ConfirmMDx

This test assesses changes that happen to your DNA when cancer cells multiply.

According to researchers, the ConfirmMDx can tell doctors which patients have truly negative biopsies and which are at higher risk. And because of that, it can reduce repeat biopsies in patients who might have otherwise received them routinely.

In a nutshell, the lab can run this test on the tissue from a biopsy. If it's negative, there's a 90 percent chance you don't have to worry. And that saves you an awful lot of unnecessary repeat biopsies. In fact, this test has been able to reduce repeat biopsies by ten-fold.

This test is available now. Some insurance plans already cover it, as does Medicare.

Two simple strategies that stop vision loss in its tracks

Age-related macular degeneration (AMD) may not be the world's leading cause of blindness. (That honor goes to cataracts.) But it's a major one, nevertheless. So it's important to know the signs. Especially if you're over 60, when most cases of AMD strike. It's even more important to know about the simple nutritional interventions that can make a *huge* difference in this disease's progression. And knowing about them might just save your eyesight in the long run.

As the name suggests, macular degeneration destroys your macula. This is the most sensitive part of your retina, located in the back part of your eye. It's filled with the light-sensing cells responsible for sharp, central vision. There are two main types of macular degeneration—dry AMD and wet AMD. The former is by far the most common, accounting for roughly 90 percent of all cases. It's a slow-moving disease that causes the critical sensory cells in your macula to break down and die.

Wet AMD, on the other hand, is marked by the growth of abnormal blood vessels beneath your macula. This results in a leakage of blood and fluid. Both of which damage the macula a lot more quickly than dry AMD. So it's fortunate that wet AMD is also the more rare form by a wide margin. But your risk of either form of the disease is higher if you're over 60, female, obese, or have heart disease. In both forms of macular degeneration, your peripheral vision remains intact. Objects right in front of you, however, will appear hazy and dull—often obscured by a single blurred or blind spot.

That's typically in the later stages, of course. Most cases of early AMD can only be detected through a comprehensive eye exam. You may notice subtle changes, like straight lines appearing crooked. Or you may not experience any symptoms at all.

Either way, now is the best time to start taking action. Which brings me back to the good news. Like I said, you can stop AMD—or at least, slow it down—with a few carefully selected nutrients. This, of course, includes supplements. And one of the most common recommendations, even among mainstream doctors, is what's known as the AREDS formulation.

The AREDS formulation is named for the National Eye Institute's Age Related Eye Disease Study. This was a 10-year clinical trial that evaluated the effectiveness of five different nutrients—vitamin C, vitamin E, beta-carotene, zinc, and copper.

Results showed that high daily doses of these nutrients can slam the brakes on AMD progression. One of the main products I use for vision preservation, EYE-BRITE,™ is based on the AREDS formulation. I recommend two tabs daily. I also administer a special IV cocktail to my patients with macular degeneration. Getting nutrients directly into your vein allows your body to tolerate doses that you could never take by mouth. It also facilitates better absorption.

My IV protocol features nutrients from the AREDS formulation (including vitamin C, zinc, and copper). But it delivers large doses of glutathione, a range of B-vitamins, and several other minerals, as well. (Namely magnesium, manganese, chromium, and selenium.)

The addition of glutathione is especially important to my IV protocol, since it isn't well absorbed through your gut. And that's a problem, because this antioxidant is by far one of the most powerful forms of natural protection your body has. Low levels of glutathione can speed up oxidative damage to the cells of your macula and lead to imbalances in ocular fluid pressure. Both of these phenomena are risk factors for AMD.

Meanwhile, research shows that B-vitamins prevent AMD-related vision loss, too. This is most likely due to their effect on homocysteine. I've mentioned homocysteine before—in particular, its link to heart disease. But the tiny blood vessels in your eyes are just as susceptible to this substance's negative effects. A steady stream of B vitamins can help to minimize this damage, which is why I've also included them in my IV protocol.

This approach isn't exclusive to my clinic. So it should be relatively easy to find a holistic practitioner who offers a similar treatment for macular degeneration. The American College for Advancement in Medicine (www.

acam.org) can help you to locate an experienced doctor in your area.

Eat your way to "younger" vision

I'm always telling my patients and readers that the right diet can go a long way in preventing disease. And my prescription for AMD is no different. As usual, sparing your vision requires eating *less* sugar. But it also means eating *more* of two key foods in particular.

The first is fish. A study of participants in the famous Nurses' Health Study and the Health Professionals Follow-up Study showed that eating more than four servings of fish per week lowers AMD risk by 35 percent.

And this was no small study, either. Researchers looked at data from over 72,000 men and women aged 50 and older, spanning over a decade. The results appeared in the *American Journal of Clinical Nutrition* in 2001.

These benefits are obviously related to the omega-3 content of fatty fish—and to its abundance of DHA in particular. So if you're not a fan of seafood, be sure to at least take a high-quality fish oil every day. (I generally recommend 3,000 mg of DHA/EPA.)

Astaxanthin is another reason I recommend fish. Astaxanthin is unusually good for the eyes because it's one of the few supplements that actually reach the retina, making it helpful for everything from eyestrain to retinopathy... even macular degeneration. A number of studies have noted how well astaxanthin improves blood flow to the retina. Just 4 mg per day is enough.

While you're at it, eat more salad. Leafy green vegetables are especially rich in lutein and zeaxanthin. And research shows that getting more of these carotenoids in your diet could cut your risk of AMD by 43 percent. That's a pretty serious perk for a side of spinach, kale, or collard greens. So feel free to serve with a heavy hand.

Clear away cataracts with this simple twice-a-day habit

As you age, the lens of your eye naturally thickens and yellows. Proteins build up and clump together, forming opaque spots on your eye's lens.

This, in turn, interferes with your eye's ability to refract light.

The end result is a cataract. And all the blurred vision, the dimness, the sensitivity to glare, and the dulling of colors that comes with it.

Free radicals—whether from excessive UV exposure or a dismal diet—speed up the process significantly. As many as half of all Americans will develop cataracts by the time they're 80 years old. Having diabetes can raise that risk by as much as 82 percent. And simply being overweight bumps the odds by more than 30 percent.

Just wearing UV-blocking sunglasses and keeping your blood sugar under control with—you guessed it!— proper diet and regular exercise could make a huge difference. But for more powerful cataract protection, there are a few key nutrients to consider.

Carnosine in particular has an outstanding reputation when it comes to cataract prevention. Its biological precursor, N-acetylcarnosine (NAC), is readily available in eye drop form that you can use twice a day. Both human and animal research points to its effectiveness in fighting cataract formation with daily use. It has even been shown to fight troublesome glare.

Carnosine is an adept free radical scavenger. It also combats glycation—the "browning" process by which sugar reacts with protein, and damages your body's tissues as a result. So really, this compound's role in preserving your eyes' health with age is a natural one.

Bilberry is another critical sight-saver that I would recommend to any at-risk patient. Like carnosine, it's a powerful antioxidant with a bunch of uses—cataract prevention is just one of them. But research shows that bilberry is particularly potent in this capacity, especially among diabetic patients.

Part of this is due to the circulatory support and collagen reinforcement that bilberry's active compounds offer the eyes. Studies show that, in addition to warding off cataracts, bilberry supplementation may help to sharpen night vision and prevent glaucoma, too.

For anyone with vision concerns, I typically recommend supplementing with 300 mg of bilberry extract daily.

I also recommend a product called EYE-BRITE™— two tabs daily. As I mentioned earlier, this formula features ample amounts of beta carotene, vitamin C, and vitamin E, along with omega-3s and several other key antioxidants.

Finally, there's French maritime pine bark extract (**Pycnogenol**®). Research shows this pine bark extract can ward off cataract formation in diabetic rats by boosting antioxidant activity in the eyes. And when combined with a low-carbohydrate diet, the protective effect is particularly profound.

I don't usually assign much value to animal studies. But as you may recall, I think everyone should be taking pine bark extract, anyway. So even if you don't have any of the classic cataract risk factors—and especially if you do—I still recommend supplementing with 50 to 100 mg of French maritime pine bark extract every day.

Slash your depression and anxiety by 72% with the rare, Indian "good mood root"

It would be nice if you could just call a time out and take off on vacation whenever you felt overwhelmed by stress. But we all know the real world doesn't work that way. The fact is, *everyone* lives with stress— some of us more than others. That's why it's so critical to find practical ways to buffer its negative effects on your body. And make no mistake. Stress *does* erode your health. So I'd like to take a moment to zero in on one of the more effective solutions.

Withania somnifera (also called ashwagandha) is a popular Ayurvedic (traditional Indian) herb, a potent antioxidant, and—bar none— one of your best bets for all-natural stress protection. That's because ashwagandha is an "adaptogen." This classification refers to its ability to help your body adapt to difficult circumstances. This could be actual physical stress, like critical illness or surgery. Or it could be mental stress, like a high-pressure job or an ugly divorce.

I won't go into the many ways that *either* form of stress can weigh down your health. I doubt I have to. If you've ever been at the mercy of your high-stress life, you already know the problems it can cause. And what makes ashwagandha so incredible is that it addresses practically all of them.

For one thing, research shows this herb offers powerful anxiety-relief without prescription drugs. In fact, one recent randomized, double-blind, placebo-controlled trial showed that taking 600 mg of ashwagandha for just 60 days could cut depression and anxiety scores by as much as 72 percent. And it could slash cortisol levels by nearly 28 percent.

This is important because chronically elevated cortisol levels can disrupt a long list of your body's vital processes. Not least of all, its immune activity. So it's hardly surprising that research supports ashwagandha as a natural immune modulator and anti-inflammatory.

I'm constantly warning about the insidious role that inflammation plays in disease development. It's a smoking gun behind arthritis, heart disease, diabetes…the list goes on. And yes, ashwagandha may help to ward off *all* of these conditions to some degree.

So for all you stressed out readers, here's my recommendation: Take 150 mg of ashwagandha, three times per day. A natural shot of relaxation is the least of what you stand to gain.

The "women's only" diet trick that reduces hot flashes by 20%

I'm a huge fan of bioidentical hormone replacement therapy. But that's just one option for menopause relief. In fact, a couple of great new studies address this very subject.

One recent study shows that simply tweaking your diet could do a number on hot flashes. Australian researchers followed a group of over 6,000 menopausal women for just under a decade. They assessed dietary patterns and menopause symptoms (night sweats and hot flashes). And Mediterranean-style eating habits cut hot flashes and night sweats by just over 20 percent.

My New Hamptons Health Miracle is very similar to the Mediterranean diet. It's rich in lean protein, fresh fruits and veggies, and healthy monounsaturated fats. It's absolutely deprivation-free. I know I've said it before, but if you make this "diet" a way of life, you really can't go wrong.

Two unexpected nutrients your bones need more of

A recent study shows two specific B vitamins are vital for your bones.

Researchers looked at X-rays of more than 2,800 women age 50 and older. And they tested their blood to see how much vitamin B, homocysteine, and various types of bone-related compounds it contained.

They found that the women who had normal bone mineral density (BMD) in their spines had higher folate levels than women who had low BMD or spinal osteoporosis. The women with osteoporosis also had higher homocysteine levels.

And the women who had low levels of B12 had a significantly higher risk of dangerously low BMD and osteoporosis.

So the solution is simple. Keep your bones healthy by getting plenty of vitamin B. Especially B12 and folate.

You can find B12 in fish, poultry, meat, and eggs. And clams and liver are loaded with it. Spinach and other dark green leafy vegetables are good sources of folate.

Of course, you should also take a high-quality vitamin B supplement. I usually recommend taking a B-100 complex each day. And to round out your bone-support regimen, you should also take 500-600 mg of calcium, 125 mg of magnesium taurate, 500 mg of strontium, 99 mg of potassium citrate, and at least 5,000 IU of vitamin D each day, as well as 5 mcg of vitamin K2 twice per day.

A natural hearing aid

You still haven't seen—or heard—everything B vitamins can do. In one study published in the *Annals of Internal Medicine*, a group of Dutch researchers recruited 728 older men and women with hearing trouble. For three years, half the group took 800 mcg folic acid daily.

At the study's end, both groups had lost some hearing. However, the folic acid group had less loss in the low-frequency range (1.0 decibel vs. 1.7 decibels).

That's right, the folic acid actually helped slow hearing loss.

Sounds like good—and simple—insurance for keeping your hearing in tip-top shape. Folic acid supplements are widely available. And it never hurts to get a little extra from food sources like spinach, asparagus, and avocado.

That could be especially important if you take certain over-the-counter pain relievers. A study out of Brigham and Women's Hospital shows that women who take ibuprofen or acetaminophen twice or more a week are at higher risk of hearing loss. And that risk rises with every extra dose you take.

So what happens if you rely on over-the-counter pain relievers six or more days per week? According to this study, your risk of hearing loss jumps by nearly 25 percent.

Researchers aren't entirely sure what's behind this association. It could be that NSAIDs decrease blood flow to the cochlea, which is the part of your inner ear that facilitates hearing. Or it could be that these popular medications simply interfere with your body's natural hearing protection mechanisms.

Whatever the reason, these findings drive home an important point. Drugs are drugs, whether they require a prescription or not. Of course their manufacturers are going to overstate their safety. But the risks of long-term use are still very real.

Your "pill-free" pooping solution

The symptoms associated with irritable bowels are *very* real. And they can have a profound impact on your quality of life.

But what most mainstream physicians call IBS is usually the symptom (or symptoms) of a deeper problem. And you can probably guess how I feel about treating symptoms without dealing with their root cause.

Simply put, it makes no sense. Yet all too often, that's just what doctors do.

This is tragic, really. Because the majority of patients who've walked into my office with an IBS diagnosis have gone on to enjoy *complete* recoveries. And all it took was targeted dietary changes and a few key nutritional supplements.

I'll get to those in a minute. First, let's take a closer look at what's really going on in your gut.

Before going any further, I'd like to note the critical difference between IBS (irritable bowel syndrome) and IBD (inflammatory bowel disease).

Simply put, IBD involves actual structural damage to the GI tract. This includes conditions like Crohn's disease and ulcerative colitis, which are accompanied by marked inflammation of the colon and which often have autoimmune roots. The IBS solutions I provide in this article will also help patients with IBD. But bear in mind that these are very different conditions. And proper diagnosis is important.

IBS, on the other hand, is a non-specific term that refers to a cluster of symptoms-namely, recurrent bouts of gas, bloating, diarrhea, or constipation. Sometimes all of the above.

To make matters worse, clinical tests have never been able to pinpoint a single cause. So as far as most mainstream physicians are concerned, in cases of IBS, your bowels are just "irritable."

But just because a colonoscopy doesn't show any digestive tract abnormalities, that doesn't mean there isn't anything going on in there. Because obviously, there *is*.

There are plenty of potential IBS triggers that a physical exam won't necessarily find.

Things like gluten intolerance. Or leaky gut, in which the lining of your digestive tract becomes irritated and permeable. (This inhibits proper nutrient absorption and introduces inflammatory elements into your bloodstream.)

Yeast overgrowth from a poorly populated digestive tract is another alarmingly common problem. And it's a major contributor to IBS. That's one of the reasons I talk about the importance of beneficial bacteria so much.

Ultimately, there are any number of potential culprits behind IBS symptoms. But pretty much all of them have the same solution.

1. It probably won't surprise you when I say that the first key to beating IBS is changing the way you eat.

But contrary to popular belief, that *doesn't* include filling up on those fancy probiotic yogurts. In fact, that's probably the *last* thing you want to put in your body. For one thing, it's usually packed with sugar—which cancels out any benefit of good bacteria.

2. Then there's the fact that dairy itself can be a major gut-irritant. So in this case, I recommend avoiding it. Many people with IBS have a difficult time digesting lactose. (That's the natural sugar in milk).

But milk proteins can also be a problem. Casein in particular-which, along with gluten and yeast, is one of the most common food sensitivities. So this is one instance where I recommend eliminating cheese, too. (Although some people find that they can tolerate it in small amounts. The only way to know for sure is to reintroduce it and watch for symptoms.)

3. It also means that bread is off the table too. Eliminating gluten is especially important. This wheat protein is easily the No. 1 cause of digestive problems of *any* kind—indigestion, GERD, bloating, gas, constipation, diarrhea, and of course, IBS.

But many of my patients have found their sensitivity to grains isn't limited to wheat. All grains—including gluten-free grains like corn and oats—contain potentially aggravating proteins that can pave the way to gut permeability. That's why eliminating all grains, and not just gluten, is often a necessity for optimal health.

Besides, whole grains are also chock-full of insoluble fiber. And too much insoluble fiber can trigger a case of the "runs" and leave you feeling bloated if you have a problem gut.

4. Unfortunately, this means that you may have to limit other healthy fiber-rich foods like leafy greens—at least until you're able to identify your own personal IBS triggers. But thoroughly cooking your vegetables can minimize these digestion difficulties, too.

5. You should also eliminate any excess sugar in your diet. Consuming excess sugar will trigger and exacerbate IBS symptoms. Again, it goes back to imbalanced gut bacteria (technically known as dysbiosis). Without enough good bacteria, certain dietary sugars—even otherwise harmless ones—are harder to digest. Extreme dysbiosis allows sugars to ferment excessively in your gut. And this can cause severe bloating, gas, and pain, among other unpleasant symptoms.

These dietary sugars fall into four specific categories—fermentable oligosaccharides, disaccharides, monosaccharides, and polyols. And there's actually a whole diet based around eliminating them, called the FODMAP diet.

The idea is to steer clear of FODMAP-rich foods. This includes obvious problem ingredients like high fructose corn syrup, agave, honey, artificial sweeteners, and sugar alcohols like sorbitol, mannitol, and xylitol.

But there are some surprising foods on the list as well. Even some healthy staples of my New Hamptons Health Miracle are packed with FODMAPs. And some IBS sufferers have to avoid them by necessity.

The complete FODMAP list is extensive, so I won't include one here. (You can get a complete rundown of FODMAP Foods on my website.) In the meantime, I put together a short list on page 43, outlining some of the FODMAP foods that would normally get a thumbs-up on my New Hamptons Health Miracle.

But if you've cleaned up your diet and are still having serious gut problems, it might be time to dig a little deeper for answers.

6. The first place I usually start is with **comprehensive allergy testing**.

In fact, this is just a good idea anyway. But be careful which kind of allergy testing you choose. Those traditional skin prick tests are notoriously unreliable.

I have all my patients get an ALCAT test, which screens for a variety of different food sensitivities based on antibody reactions from a blood sample.

I recommend the "100 Food Panel" at a minimum. But the more comprehensive the panel, the better, if you can afford it. (All of these tests are relatively pricey—but in my opinion, absolutely worth it.)

You don't even have to see a doctor for ALCAT testing. You can order one online at www.alcat.com or by calling 1-800-872-5228. They will send someone to you directly to draw your blood sample then overnight it to the lab. Then they will help you find a doctor in your area to review the results or provide a wellness advisor.

Obviously, if your ALCAT test turns up specific food sensitivities, you should cut those items from your diet (along with dairy, grains, and sugar as I recommended above).

There are a lot of other factors that can aggravate IBS issues—like stress levels, hormones, you name it. But the culprits I mentioned above are by far some of most common. And whatever the cause of your IBS, dietary changes will absolutely make a difference.

7. So will upping your intake of a few nutrients in particular.

There are lots of supplements you can take to keep IBS under control. And you might have to experiment a little to find a combo that best suits your particular symptoms. (Working with a physician skilled in natural medicine will help streamline the process. If you don't already have a naturopathic doctor, you can find one in your area by contacting the American College for Advancement in Medicine at 800-532-3688 or www.acam.org.)

That said, there are a few supplements I recommend to everyone dealing with irritable bowels. The first, is a high-quality **probiotic** like Dr. Ohhira's.

The second, which might be slightly more surprising, is **vitamin D**. Preliminary research shows that high-dose vitamin D can deliver significant improvements to IBS symptoms. Anecdotal reports peg the success rate around 70 percent.

That certainly reflects my experience—which makes pretty good odds for a nutrient that you really should be taking anyway.

I always recommend at least 2,000 to 5,000 IUs of vitamin D3 every day—but you can safely take up to 10,000 IUs. And in the winter, when sun exposure is minimal, this might be necessary.

I also advise taking regular doses of **pantethine (B5)**—1,500 mg, three times per day. This serves a dual purpose. On one hand, it helps your body process the toxic byproducts of Candida overgrowth (namely a chemical called acetaldehyde), which happen to spike in your body when the yeast begins to die off.

This is, of course, a *good* thing. But it can have unpleasant side effects—also known as the Herxheimer reaction. Symptoms can include headaches, fatigue, digestive upset, muscle or joint pain, flu-like

Fifteen healthy foods that could be wreaking havoc on your bowels

This list might surprise you. And, yes, these are all foods that are included in my New Hamptons Health Miracle. The fact is, there's nothing inherently "wrong" with any of them. In fact, they can offer tremendous health benefits for most people. But if you've got IBS, they can make your symptoms a lot worse. So you'll feel a whole lot better if you avoid them and stick with the other delicious choices included in my New Hamptons Health Miracle. (Don't worry—there are plenty of them!)

If you have IBS, avoid the following FODMAP foods:

Artichokes	Cauliflower	Onions
Avocado	Garlic	Pistachios
Asparagus	Green beans	Summer squash
Broccoli	Leeks	Watermelon
Brussels sprouts	Mushrooms	
Cabbage	Okra	

symptoms, and rashes.

Simply put, you'll feel worse before you feel better. (Sometimes a lot worse.) But pantethine can help minimize this reaction.

As an added bonus, pantethine also boosts adrenal function. This is important because stress can paralyze your bowels, which renders them unable to process your food. And what happens? Your meals "go right through you," so to speak.

Vitamin A is another staple for my patients dealing with IBS. I recommend 40,000 IU of vitamin A per day. You need plenty of vitamin A to reinforce the junctions of your intestinal walls and ensure proper function of the cells lining your gut. So needless to say, deficiencies can have serious consequences for gut barrier function.

This is the same reason I advise anyone struggling with IBS to fill up on a combo of gut-strengthening botanicals and other nutrients. Along with vitamin A, they can help heal leaky gut and strengthen the mucosal lining of your digestive tract.

Which is especially important after years of dealing with one or more undiagnosed food sensitivities.

Obviously, it's easier if you can find a product that combines these nutrients into a single formula. (Any comprehensive GI support product will feature several or all of them.) But either way, the dosages I shoot for are generally as follows:

- Deglycyrrhized licorice (DGL)—500 mg per day
- Aloe vera leaf extract—250 mg per day
- N-acetyl glucosamine—250 mg per day
- Slippery elm bark—200 mg per day
- Marshmallow root—100 mg per day

So there you have it. My foolproof prescription for healthy bowels.

In fact, go ahead and call it a cure. Because I'm willing to bet that, like so many of my patients, your results with this combination of strategies will be just that powerful. And most importantly, permanent.

Lose 35% more weight with the fat-fighting antioxidant you've never heard of

There's no getting around it. Losing weight can be hard. But more and more research shows that one of the most important things you can do when you're cutting calories is to take alpha lipoic acid (ALA).

ALA is one of my all-time favorite dietary supplements. This antioxidant is a powerhouse for heart, liver, and kidney health. And it can help control blood sugar and fight diabetes.

ALA is especially important when you're dieting, for two reasons:

- It enhances your body's ability to convert food into energy.
- It discourages fat formation.

And now a new study confirms that it can help you lose significantly more weight than dieting alone. ALA can do this by itself or combined with another all-star, eicosapentaenoic acid. EPA is one of the primary essential omega-3 fatty acids found in fish oil.

In the 10-week study, 97 overweight or obese women were put on an eating plan in which their total daily calories were cut by 30 percent. The women were then divided into four groups. One group was given 300 mg of ALA daily, one group received 1.3 grams of EPA a day, and another group was given both ALA and EPA. The fourth group got a placebo.

At the end of the study, the placebo group lost an average of 11.4 pounds, and the EPA group lost an average of 11.9 pounds.

The women who took ALA lost the most weight—a whopping 15.4 pounds on average. The ALA/EPA group was close behind, losing 14.3 pounds.

While the group taking ALA lost the most weight, researchers said the EPA supplementation significantly reduced the decrease in leptin, the hormone that regulates hunger.

So if hunger pangs derail your weight-loss efforts, you might want to supplement your ALA regimen with EPA. You'll lose almost as much weight and likely feel more comfortable doing it.

I recommend taking 100 mg of ALA three times a day. It's an easy way to be slimmer and healthier overall.

And if you want to add EPA, I recommend taking it in the form of fish oil so that you get a dose of the essential fatty acid DHA at the same time. I typically recommend 3,000 mg EPA and DHA per day.

The "apple and cheese" secret that can help you live 25% longer

I recently uncovered new research on a natural supplement that could help you live longer…and better. It's called oxaloacetate (or OAA). It may sound like some sort of chemical concocted in a lab, but I can assure you OAA is totally natural. Also known as oxaloacetic acid, it's found in apples, dairy products, and fermented foods like yogurt and red wine.

1. Get energized at the cellular level

The body uses OAA to help produce energy at a cellular level. Basically, OAA helps your cells make a substance called adenosine triphosphate, or ATP. And ATP provides the basic energy every cell in your body needs to do its job—whether it's digesting your breakfast or remembering the name of your sixth-grade teacher.

Unfortunately, as you age, your cells don't produce ATP as well as they once did. But researchers are learning that you can reverse that energy drain if you have enough of the components your body needs to make ATP—especially OAA. In fact, one study showed that depriving cells of OAA can cause their energy production to fall by a whopping 500%.

2. Defend your brain

Researchers have discovered OAA can help flush a neurotransmitter called glutamate out of your body. You need glutamate for learning and memory, but when you have too much, it can become toxic, killing off brain cells. Stress can send glutamate levels soaring, and studies have found too much glutamate can also encourage cancer cells to grow.

Research shows OAA can flush excess glutamate from your brain in as little as 90 minutes.

Plus, one recent study shows that OAA has a triple whammy effect directly on brain cells—it helps promote cell energy, reduce inflammation, and actually create new cells.

Two independent clinical studies also show that OAA's ability to reduce glutamate can significantly improve neurological performance and function in people who have had a stroke.

3. Live 25% longer

OAA has even been proven to mimic the longevity benefits of calorie restriction…without actually having to cut calories. Restricting calories is one of the best known ways to increase lifespan, but it can also help fight off serious diseases like cancer, Alzheimer's, Parkinson's, and diabetes.

In a study on worms, researchers found that OAA can have the same effects, but without reducing calories. In fact, the worms given OAA lived an average of 25% longer than those that didn't take OAA.

There have been other OAA longevity trials on animals that show equally impressive results. Of course, none of this is the same as research on people. But because humans live so long, a study on OAA's longevity effects will take decades before it's finished. In the meantime, the animal research appears quite promising.

4. Fight cancer 237% more effectively

Glutamate can play a role in the growth of malignant brain tumors known as gliomas. And it also helps other types of cancer cells grow and divide. So it makes sense that by reducing the levels of glutamate in your body, OAA can help you fight the development and spread of cancer.

In fact, research shows that mice with gliomas that were given OAA had a 237% better survival rate than the ones not given OAA.

How much OAA do you need and where can you find it?

OAA can be found in certain foods, but only in small amounts—not the 100—250 mg daily that's been proven in studies to be effective. That's why I recommend OAA supplements.

There are only a few companies that market OAA supplements. If you can't find it at your local nutritional supplement store, you can buy it online.

Look for formulas that use thermally stabilized OAA because OAA is notoriously volatile. If it's not thermally stabilized, it has to be stored at ultra-freezing temperatures to ensure it stays safe and effective. OAA is usually combined with vitamin C, which helps further stabilize it.

How a bit of "gold dust" slashes blood sugar, blood pressure, cholesterol, and diarrhea

Centuries ago in China, village doctors used a simple herbal remedy to treat one of their most devastating illnesses—a lethal form of diarrhea known as dysentery. They also used this remedy to treat what they referred to as "Wasting-Thirst Syndrome." Today, we know it better as Type 2 diabetes.

But, in those very primitive times—long before donuts and delivery pizza—dysentery was an even bigger killer than diabetes. Over time, its blood sugar effects faded into obscurity, and it became known as THE cure for diarrhea…for stomach upsets of all kinds, in fact.

Fast-forward to the 1980s, when a team of researchers accidentally re-discovered its diabetes-defeating potential…

What is this ancient healing miracle?

The Traditional Chinese Doctors called it Zhi Mu, but today it's more commonly known as berberine, which translates as "golden thread."

The modern-day rediscovery of berberine's blood sugar potential began in 1983 in a hospital in northeast China. A local doctor, Ni Yanxi, was treating several patients for diarrhea…patients who also had diabetes. As expected, berberine took care of the patients' stomach issues.

But much to Ni Yanxi's surprise, something else happened too…

All of his patients' blood sugar levels had gone down significantly.

He re-tested his results to make sure he was right. Once again, berberine brought down subjects' blood sugar—this time by a whopping 86%, with effects that started in as little as an hour after taking it.

And with that, the diabetes-defeating potential for berberine was re-born. Over the past 29 years, study after study—conducted in the best laboratories all over the world—have proven berberine's amazing blood sugar balancing powers. In fact, clinical trials indicate that…

This "golden thread" stands up to the mainstream's "gold-standard" treatment

In one study, again conducted in China, researchers put berberine to the test against Metformin, one of the most widely prescribed blood sugar drugs.

The researchers were blown away to find that in both groups...

- Hemoglobin A1c fell by 2 percent
- Post-meal blood sugar levels plummeted by more than 8 points
- Insulin resistance dropped by one third

Researchers even called the results "identical"! And all of these benefits began after just one week.

The biggest diabetes breakthrough of the 21st century?

It's easy to be skeptical when one substance seems to "do it all"... and scientists are. But their studies have started to unlock some of berberine's healing secrets.

Research has revealed a new understanding of how diabetes develops. Scientists believe that diabetes is caused by a low-grade inflammation (as is high cholesterol, high blood pressure, and other chronic diseases).

And that's how many Traditional Chinese Medicine remedies work— they quiet inflammation, bringing the body's internal mechanisms into balance. Studies show it takes just a bit of berberine to ease this inflammation, and, in turn, to get blood sugar into check.

But there's still more to the story. Let me back up a step and explain just how...

Berberine attacks the root of the problem

A group of scientists in Haikou, China, have come up with a hypothesis on the link between inflammation and blood sugar problems. And, believe it or not, they pinpoint an imbalance in gut bacteria as the culprit.

Their research, published in the July 2011 issue of *Medical Science Monitor* suggests that an imbalance in gut bacteria causes the low-grade inflammation that, in turn, leads to diabetes.

When the imbalance is corrected, diabetes doesn't develop.

And these researchers believe that berberine has significant power to kill bad bacteria, thus reducing inflammation…and balancing blood sugar.

Now, there's some compelling scientific evidence that berberine also helps promote weight loss.

Researchers gave participants 500 milligrams of berberine three times a day for 12 weeks. By the end of the study, the subjects had lost an average of about 5 pounds per person. They also had a 23 percent decrease in triglycerides.

Previous studies by the same researchers showed that berberine actually prevents fat accumulation.

Plus, researchers discovered yet another surprising benefit of berberine. The study participants also had a whopping 59.5% increase in their levels of vitamin D3 (the active form of the vitamin, also known as calcitriol levels). The researchers concluded that this makes berberine a contender for maintaining healthy bone density.

There were no indications of safety problems from taking berberine. All the standard heart, liver, and kidney function tests came out fine.

Fight for your health with food—and beat back blood sugar for good

In 1822, it took the average American five days to consume the amount of sugar you'll find in a single 12-ounce can of soda. Today, most people consume that much sugar every 7 hours. And the real reason behind our country's skyrocketing rate of chronic disease is clear as day. Sugar kills—it's as simple as that.

So if you really want to get a jump on liver and blood-sugar health, you've got to give up starchy, sugary foods. And soda and other sweetened drinks, in particular.

Stick strictly to lean proteins, veggies, healthy fats, eggs, cheese, and low sugar fruits (like berries and melon). And you will have already taken the single most important step towards ultimate liver and blood-sugar health there is.

When I first saw the research on berberine I knew I had to use it at my office.

I started out with my most troublesome patients, and, wouldn't you know—in all five of them, blood sugar decreased so much I actually needed to lower their medications (which is why it's important to work with your doctor if you decide to take berberine).

Since then I've used berberine in all of my patients with diabetes and blood sugar problems—and in the overweight patients—with incredible success.

In fact, I would venture to say that berberine has changed my practice more significantly than any nutrient I can remember.

I recommend starting with 500 mg of berberine per day, and monitoring the effect on your blood sugar. You can safely increase the dose gradually, up to 1,500 mg per day—until you reach the optimum blood sugar level.

The secret to bringing your blood sugar down as much as 28%—in mere minutes

A recent study showed that a quick workout can lead to some major improvements in your blood sugar. Here's how it works...

Researchers had a group of sedentary people do three of these workouts a week for six weeks. Each workout consisted of easy cycling and sprinting.

The first week, the subjects only sprinted once during their 10-minute workout. And only for 10 seconds.

The next two weeks, they sprinted twice during the routine. Each sprint lasted 15 seconds.

The last three weeks, they continued with two sprints per workout. But those sprints were each 20 seconds long.

At the end of six weeks, these short workouts led to a whopping 28 percent improvement in insulin function.

I know what you're thinking. "Dr. Fred, I can't even jog, let alone sprint." But hear me out...

We're not talking about long distances here. Or even a lot of time. In fact, these "sprinting" workouts only last 10 minutes. Total. That's even less time than the 15-minute after-dinner walk I ask all my patients to commit to. And you only have to sprint for 20 seconds—max.

It's certainly well worth a try for such an impressive result.

Chapter 4

The natural prescription for a PAIN-FREE life

Migraines. Arthritis. Back pain. They couldn't be more different, right?

Actually, they're more similar than you may think. In fact, they all boil down to one, single underlying cause...

Inflammation.

Of course Big Pharma has made billions selling the idea that all the different types of pain require a different bottle in your medicine cabinet.

Tylenol Back Pain...Advil Arthritis...Excedrin Migraine—the list is endless. But really, they all address pain the same way. By relieving inflammation.

Problem is, their effects are only temporary. So as soon as they wear off, the inflammation—and your pain—comes back.

But here's a little secret those drug makers don't want you to know...

You CAN get rid of pain and inflammation entirely—with just a few simple steps. And it's important to do so, because left unchecked, inflammation can be killer.

In itself, inflammation is a good thing. It's how your body protects itself. And how it heals itself. Without it, wounds and infections would never get better.

Here's how it works. Any time you injure yourself or are exposed to some sort of infection, your immune system responds by sending out substances called "inflammatory mediators." Histamine, prostaglandins, and cytokines are probably the most well-known.

The inflammatory mediators increase blood flow. They also allow more white blood cells to get through your blood vessel walls to the site of the infection or injury.

All of this is necessary to heal you. But in the process, it can also cause redness, fever, swelling, and—yes—**pain**.

This sort of response is known as acute *inflammation*. And it generally goes away on its own within a few days (at the most).

But when it doesn't go away, it results in something called *chronic inflammation*. Which causes ongoing pain (among other symptoms)—and generally makes your life miserable.

This sort of inflammation is at the root of arthritis pain, fibromyalgia, back pain, etc. And if you don't rein it in, it can lead to more serious conditions.

Research has linked chronic inflammation to heart disease, cancer, and Alzheimer's disease.

But as complicated as the inflammatory process is, keeping it under control is actually quite simple. And like most health problems, the best place to start battling inflammation is with food.

I believe there's a simple reason arthritis, back aches, and so many other forms of pain are at record highs these days. It all comes back to the dreadful diet that's become the "standard" in this country.

You see, the Standard American Diet relies heavily on packaged, processed foods. And these contain large amounts of omega-6 fatty acids. I've talked before about the importance of fatty acids. But even more important than fatty acids themselves is the ratio of fatty acids in your body.

Omega-6s are generally known as "pro-inflammatory" fatty acids. So you need to balance them out with other essential fatty acids to neutralize this effect. Otherwise, your body is in a constant state of inflammation. And you're much more likely to suffer from ongoing aches and pains.

And being overweight—which is also much more likely if you're eating a lot of packaged, processed carbs—compounds the inflammation problem even more. Body fat, especially belly fat, triggers a low-grade inflammatory process throughout the body. Studies show that people with chronic low-grade inflammation have two to three times the levels of inflammatory markers such as TNF-a, IL-6, and C-Reactive protein.

To put it simply, immune cells mistake fatty deposits as intruders. When fat cells expand and leak, your body releases more inflammatory chemicals. It's a vicious cycle. But there's an easy solution...

Cut out the processed, packaged foods. Instead, focus on whole, natural, minimally processed foods.

That single, simple step alone will make a huge difference in easing inflammation throughout your body. In fact, it will probably get you most of the way there without doing anything else.

And it's not as difficult as it might seem to make the switch. You've probably heard this advice before, but shopping the "perimeter" of the grocery store is the simplest way to bypass most processed foods altogether. (Avoid "foods" like crackers, granola bars, cereals, bottled salad dressings, etc. All the products that fill up the center aisles in the supermarket.) Stock your shopping cart with vegetables, fruit, cheese, meat, and seafood. Another good option is to do as much food shopping at your local farmers' market as you can. Not only are the foods you'll find there unprocessed, but they're also more likely to be organic, are locally grown, and seasonal. So you can be sure they're truly healthy. (Plus, they taste better, too.)

My New Hamptons Health Miracle makes it simple—and delicious—to cut out the processed foods that contribute to chronic inflammation.

In the meantime, there are also a few supplements that can help you get even better results...

Fish oil. This is the best source of the omega-3 fatty acids EPA (eicosapentaenoic acid) and DHA (docosahexaenoic acid). Studies show that omega-3s have powerful anti-inflammatory effects. And you need plenty of omega-3s to balance out those pro-inflammatory omega-6s. For fish oil supplements, check the label for the EPA/DHA content. This is the most important part of any fish oil supplement. And you want to get the most bang for your buck. You need 3,000 mg of EPA/DHA (not just fish oil) per day.

Vitamin D. Two new studies show how important vitamin D is for pain and inflammation. The first study, published in *The Journal of Immunology*, showed that vitamin D is directly related to how well your body handles inflammation. Based on their findings, the researchers concluded that people with low levels of vitamin D aren't able to regulate inflammation. But people whose levels are within the normal range can keep inflammation from raging out of control and contributing to problems like asthma, arthritis, and cancer.

The second study was even more impressive. Researchers looked at 2,070 adults over age 65. More than half—53 percent—reported having moderate to severe pain. Every single one also had low vitamin D levels. Just 10 minutes of sun exposure daily is all it takes. But if you're wearing sunscreen, you probably aren't getting sufficient amounts. That's where supplements are essential. I recommend at least 2,000-5,000 IU per day of vitamin D3. And be sure to get your blood levels checked periodically by your physician. It should be in the 50+ range.

Bromelain. This pineapple extract is best known in the natural medicine world as a digestive enzyme. But it also has powerful anti-inflammatory effects. In fact, in 2008 Duke University researchers found that bromelain can decrease migration of white blood cells to sites of acute inflammation. A dose of 200 mg per day is usually plenty.

MSM. This sulfur compound has been around in supplement form for a long time. Most of the evidence supporting its powerful pain-relieving effects is anecdotal. But in 2009, a Korean study showed that MSM does inhibit a number of inflammatory mediators. I generally recommend 2,000 mg three times per day.

CoEnzyme Q10 (CoQ10). On its own CoQ10 has some solid research supporting its ability to reduce inflammation. But a new study conducted at the University of Cordoba in Spain made an interesting discovery. You can get even more anti-inflammatory benefits when you add CoQ10 to a diet based on lean protein, fruits, vegetables, and monounsaturated fatty acids. (Sound familiar?)

Researchers found that the diet alone made a big dent in curbing participants' inflammation. But when they took 200 mg of CoQ10 too, they got even better results.

One more reason to get moving

I know. When you're in pain, exercise is the last thing you want to think about. But it's actually one of the best things you can do to overcome it.

Research has shown that regular physical activity decreases markers of inflammation. Activity also releases endorphins, the brain chemicals that improve a person's mood, which simply helps you cope better. And exercise will help you lose weight, which helps ease inflammation even further. Plus, it takes some excess stress off your knees and hips, and that helps relieve back pain.

I advise my patients to start with stretching and muscle strengthening exercises. You'll be surprised what a big difference it can make. But don't stop once your pain starts to subside!

You need to keep moving—and keep eating healthy foods and taking the right supplements—to keep those anti-inflammatory, pain-relieving benefits going.

Relief for acute flare-ups

Of course, even if you've taken every step outlined above to protect yourself from chronic inflammation and pain, every now and then you're bound to have an acute flare-up. Whether it's a headache, a bruise, or sore muscles from overdoing it in the garden. So here are some of my go-to recommendations for nipping acute pain in the bud.

Arnica. This herbal, homeopathic remedy has been used for more than 500 years to treat pain and inflammation. But it's got some modern science behind it as well.

One study looked at 204 people with osteoarthritis in their hands. Researchers found that a topical arnica gel worked just as well as ibuprofen for relieving pain. You can use topical arnica creams. Or you can look for homeopathic sublingual tablets (in the 30x potency). If you opt for tablets, I recommend 5 under the tongue five times per day.

White willow bark. This is Nature's aspirin. In fact, aspirin is actually a synthetic form of salicin, the natural compound in white willow bark. But the natural form is much, much safer. I typically recommend 400 mg tablets up to four times per day.

Curcumin. This extract comes from the spice turmeric. One study found that 2 grams of curcumin extract provides pain relief similar to ibuprofen.

Capsaicin. This hot pepper extract stimulates circulation, desensitizes nerve endings, and acts as a local anesthetic. It's usually used topically. And studies have shown it's very effective for many different types of pain with few—if any—side effects.

A sure-fire fix that turns "useless" arthritis remedies into miracle cures

Maybe you've tried natural arthritis remedies before. And maybe you've had less-than-stellar results.

There are certainly plenty of reports to back up your experience. In fact, you hear more stories claiming that natural arthritis remedies don't work than ones claiming they DO.

But before you write them off altogether, consider this…

None of those supplement-bashing stories ever talk about WHY natural arthritis remedies don't live up to expectations.

But after decades of research and hands-on experience with my patients, I've finally pieced this mystery together. There's a hidden reason so many people never seem to be able to get the arthritis relief they so desperately need.

It turns out, you may actually have a problem with your STOMACH!

You see, every nutrient that supports your joints must pass through your stomach first. And if your stomach isn't operating up to par… Well, you may not get all the healing potential those natural remedies really have to offer.

Problem is, it's not always so easy to tell if your digestion is out of whack. But here's a quick checklist of some things that can throw it off kilter. Do you…

- Chew your food too quickly?
- Eat on the run?
- Eat junk food?
- Eat late in the day?
- Drink alcohol?

If any of these apply to you (and, let's be honest—they apply to most of us), chances are good your stomach isn't quite at the top of its game.

And, unfortunately your joints may be paying the price.

But start with your stomach, and before you know it, those natural arthritis remedies will go from useless to miraculous.

Bromelain (from pineapple) and **papain** (from papaya) are two common, widely available digestive enzymes that can help your body break down arthritis-relieving supplements and use them more effectively.

Pancreatin and **pepsin** are two other options I often recommend to my patients.

Of course, it's always best to work with a doctor to find the right combination and dose. To find a natural physician near you who will be familiar with digestive enzymes, contact the American College for Advancement in Medicine at www.acam.org.

But, rest assured, in many cases, all it takes is a few of these specific enzymes to jumpstart your digestion. And—*voila!* You unlock all the healing potential inside those natural joint supplements. Which means you'll finally get that relief you've been searching for.

How to wipe out arthritis pain—and a whole lot more—without a single drug

Enzymes are the catalysts behind every single important event that takes place in your body. Like a finger pushing an intricate line of dominos, these tiny molecules set off the chain of events that make life itself possible.

In fact, there's a theory out there that the length of your life is directly related to your body's enzyme status. And that the state of your health rests on the shoulders of these vital molecules.

This same theory suggests that simply supplementing with enzymes can lead to a longer, healthier life.

But could perfect health *really* be that easy?

Well, I'm not sure I'd go quite that far. There are other factors involved in longevity that are equally important (a healthy diet and regular exercise being two of the most obvious).

But I do know that enzymes are incredibly underused in modern medicine. And it's absolutely true that your health depends on them—in more ways than you might think.

> ## Five telltale signs of enzyme deficiency
>
> How do you know if you're lacking critical enzymes? If you're over 40, it's practically inevitable. But here are five telltale signs of enzyme deficiency:
>
> - heartburn
> - bloating and gas
> - food sensitivities
> - fatigue
> - aches and pains
>
> If any of these symptoms sound familiar, a digestive enzyme supplement is definitely in order.

Benefits way beyond your stomach

The most common uses of enzymes revolve around digestion. I frequently recommend enzymes to patients with nausea, diarrhea, ulcers, GERD, or hiatal hernias. But I also use them for patients suffering from conditions that don't have anything to do with digestion—like serious injuries or joint pain.

And there's a good reason for that.

Enzymes are responsible for breaking down the food you eat into vitamins and minerals that your body can actually use for nutrition.

But enzymes also go way beyond that.

At the most basic level, enzymes are proteins that make life-sustaining chemical reactions happen. They're what keep the complex clockwork of your cells, organs, bones, muscles, and every other conceivable living tissue running.

Unfortunately, you lose enzymes as you age. Take the enzyme that converts the omega-3 ALA into the active forms of EPA and DHA, for example. In most people, it's gone by age 40.

It's a sinister sequence of events. One that essentially paves the way toward disease—and even death. And there are a few factors that make the problem even worse.

How you eat is just as important as *what* you eat

First of all, your levels of stomach acid start to decline with age. And stomach acid is partially responsible for activating your digestive enzymes.

In a perfect world, your food would pick up most of the slack caused by this natural decline. Fresh, raw food is packed with live enzymes that help to maximize nutrient absorption. But "fresh" and "raw" are the key words here.

Obviously, processed foods are about as far from nature—and devoid of life-sustaining enzymes—as it gets.

But when I say "fresh," I mean food that just came out of the ground or off the tree. The enzymes in fruits and vegetables start to degrade the moment you harvest them. And produce that isn't local and seasonal often spends weeks in crates on a truck before it actually makes it to the supermarket.

And simply *cooking* your food strips it of vital enzymes even further. Not that I'm advocating a strictly raw food diet. But incorporating some raw or very lightly steamed or sautéed produce into your diet is always a good thing.

Then there's the rushed way so many Americans eat. You see, chewing is a vital part of the digestive process. It triggers the release of enzymes that help to break down your food. (That's why I don't recommend chewing gum—why waste precious enzymes on non-nutritive junk?)

So eating processed, enzyme-deficient food too quickly is the worst possible scenario for your body. You miss out on the important pre-digestion that occurs with thorough chewing. And the food itself doesn't contain enough enzymes to aid with digestion once it gets to your stomach.

This leaves your pancreas to generate all the enzymes necessary to eke out even a scrap of nutrition from the meal you just ate.

It's an enormous amount of pressure to put on one organ. Especially one that plays other critical roles in the body (namely insulin production and blood sugar control). This extra burden may be one reason why so many people in this country have pre-diabetes and diabetes.

So let's talk about how to tackle this uniquely modern health crisis...

The bedtime cure for leaky gut

For best results, I recommend taking a dose of whatever enzyme supplement you choose before bed, too. Because enzymes that aren't tied up with digestion will eventually make their way into your bloodstream— where they go after any undigested food particles that may have slipped through. (The byproduct of a condition called leaky gut syndrome.)

Food particles that escape through a leaky gut are targeted as foreign invaders by your immune system. And it attacks them just as it would any other threat—by triggering inflammation throughout your body (and all the problems that come with it).

So taking digestive enzymes at bedtime on an empty stomach helps combat this increasingly common problem before it even has a chance to start.

Six enzymes you need with every meal

Your first step should be to get as many live enzymes from your food as you can. As I said above, fresh, local, seasonal produce is your very best source of enzymes. And cook your vegetables just until they're ever-so-slightly tender.

You can cover the rest of your bases with a comprehensive enzyme supplement.

This is really one recommendation everyone can benefit from. Because even young, healthy people are borrowing from Peter to pay Paul (so to speak) if they're not eating a near-perfect diet.

If your enzyme reserves are limited, your body uses them for digestion first. Which means you don't have as many left for the other critical functions enzymes help carry out in your body.

This is why I often recommend enzyme supplements to treat conditions that, on the surface at least, seem to have nothing to do with digestion. Like bacterial and viral infections, and conditions associated with inflammation, including heart disease, multiple sclerosis, and cancer—just to name a few.

So here's a quick list of some of the key digestive enzymes you should be taking with every meal:

- Papain—From papaya and helps digest proteins
- Amylase—Aids the digestion of starches and carbohydrates
- Lipase—Aids the digestion of fats
- Cellulase—Helps break down fiber
- Lactase—Helps break down milk sugars in dairy products
- Bromelain—From pineapples and helps digest protein

The good news is, there are numerous products on the market that include most—if not all—of these enzymes in one formula. Even better, enzyme supplements are easy to find (your local GNC and Vitamin Shoppe likely carry several good options to choose from), and they're affordable.

You should start with a low dose and take it with every meal. Follow this prescription, and you can count on some pretty transformative results.

For one thing, you'll be giving your overburdened digestive system some much needed relief, while maximizing nutrient uptake from your food. And that's a sure path to higher energy and stronger immunity. Not to mention one of the most surprising benefits of enzyme therapy...

Arthritis relief that rivals painkilling drugs

As I mentioned above, enzymes are actually one of the most powerful weapons in your arthritis arsenal. But when it comes to tackling joint pain, one particular type of enzyme is especially important.

Let me explain: Nutrient uptake is the domain of digestive enzymes, which come from your pancreas, your stomach, your salivary glands, and ideally, your food. But any condition outside of your gut needs help from metabolic enzymes to heal.

Metabolic enzymes come almost entirely from your pancreas, with two notable exceptions: papain and bromelain, which come from food sources. They also function as both digestive and metabolic enzymes.

And that's why they're such great natural anti-inflammatories. Because like other metabolic enzymes, they have the unique ability to cruise through your blood stream and eat up foreign proteins. Not just rogue food particles but also viruses, bacteria, and—perhaps most importantly—fibrin.

Fibrin is a key player in your body's inflammatory response. And left unchecked, it can cause a lot of problems.

You may have heard about its role in the formation of deadly blood clots and heart attacks. However, fibrin deposits in the joints are also one of the defining traits of arthritis. But metabolic enzymes (like bromelain and papain) are able to dissolve them.

This probably sounds a little too good to be true. But it's not. In fact, published research shows that metabolic enzymes rival drug therapy when it comes to relieving arthritis pain and improving mobility.

Several clinical trials from the last two decades show that specialized enzyme supplementation offers the same clinical benefit as non-steroidal anti-inflammatory drugs (NSAIDs) for patients suffering with osteoarthritis of the knee.

And a 2006 study featuring patients with osteoarthritis of the hip showed similar results. This six-week study pitted enzyme therapy against a NSAID called diclofenac. And it found no significant difference in pain, stiffness, or physical function between the two treatment groups.

In fact, the results of this study leaned pretty definitively in favor of enzyme supplementation. Just over 71 percent of the patients taking enzymes showed either a good or very good response—versus 61.4 percent of the patients taking the NSAID.

And of course, enzymes are much safer than any of the NSAIDs on the market.

After all, *enzymes* certainly aren't causing heart attacks, stroke, hearing loss, or any of the other horrors you hear about on the nightly news. No—that distinction goes to NSAIDs.

So researchers may call the two arthritis treatments "equivalent." But when you factor in safety, enzymes are the clear winner.

"Maori gold": The lost solution for arthritis pain *found and forgotten* on the coast of New Zealand over 35 years ago!

You probably know New Zealand as a tiny island on the other side of the world. But hidden on its remote shores is the secret to not only soothing your arthritis pain but possibly *healing* the damaged cartilage in your joints…

According to New Zealand folklore (and now science!), eating one type of shellfish—called a **green-lipped mussel**—will help keep your joints strong, smooth and healthy well into your golden years.

The green-lipped mussel only grows naturally along the glimmering Maori coast of New Zealand. And it remained a local Maori secret until the 1960s, when western researchers stumbled upon it while searching for a cancer cure.

Unfortunately, the green-lipped mussel didn't cure cancer. But during testing, the researchers found something almost as valuable for millions suffering from *arthritis*.

A unique oil containing one of the most fascinating combinations of anti-inflammatories known to man…I like to call it, "Maori gold."

Once scientists realized this green-lipped mussel was the key to the Maori's joint comfort, it quickly led to a flood of studies. Now with more than 25 trials, scientists agree the green-lipped mussel could be your ticket to pain-free joints.

One study showed that 1,050 mg of green lipped mussel extract was able to improve joint comfort, mobility and stiffness in 76% of participants.

Another showed that 83% of participants reported good or excellent results after using 1,500 mg of green lipped mussel extract daily over a year-long period…the patients described exercising with ease, improved joint comfort, and greater mobility. Just like the Maori.

"Maori gold" even showed the ability to repair and replace damaged joint cartilage for some of the study participants. After four decades of testing, researchers now believe that the "natural compounds" responsible for the effects were the omega-3 fatty acids found in the green-lipped mussel. And what's more, as it turns out...green-lipped mussels have them in droves!

In fact, the green-lipped mussels contain more omega-3s than just about any other fish on the planet. They also contain a unique combination of fatty acids you'd be hard pressed to find in any other food.

What's their secret? Green-lipped mussels feed on a unique species of plankton that migrate to the New Zealand coast from subarctic waters.

These unique plankton contain loads of anti-inflammatory compounds that protect them from harmful ozone damage above the subarctic circle.

When green-lipped mussels eat the plankton, they inherit this ingenious defense mechanism. As a result, the green-lipped mussels contain a powerful combination of fatty acids and anti-inflammatories that are hard to find anywhere else in the world!

I know there are huge concerns about the purity of omegas. And with good reason. But green-lipped mussels are about as pure as they come. They grow in pristine waterways that are remote and government-protected off the coast of New Zealand.

So you can take green-lipped mussel extract with confidence. And enjoy not just the soothing anti-inflammatory effects, but also the potential to actually help "regenerate" the connective tissue in your joints for longer-term benefits.

I generally recommend 1,000-1,500 mg per day in capsule form.

The hidden culprit behind stubborn, aching joints in 4 out of 5 people

You already know that carrying excess pounds can put incredible strain on your joints. But here's something you probably don't know: Groundbreaking new research reveals another key factor involved in joint pain.

It's a strange hormone in your joints called leptin—which is produced by fat cells. Simply put, leptin is your body's natural way of regulating your appetite and managing your weight if you occasionally overeat.

So you'd think that loading up on leptin would help shrink your waistline, right? Unfortunately, that's not the way it works.

Researchers have discovered that people with a high body mass index (BMI) can actually have high levels of leptin. It's called leptin resistance, meaning their brain doesn't receive leptin's signal to shut down appetite. And they just keep eating—producing more fat and more leptin.

As it turns out, this hormone doesn't just control your hunger and impact your BMI... It can also dictate how healthy your joints are going to be.

How "Leptin Overload" is taking its toll on your joints

New reports from journals like *International Orthopaedics, Life Sciences,* and *Rheumatology* all confirm that too much leptin can cause:

- Thin, weak cartilage
- Supercharged inflammation
- More aches and pains in your joints

Research has revealed that 4 out of 5 people with joint pain have excess levels of leptin—or as I call it, "Leptin Overload"—in their joints. Specifically, studies show that people who carry extra weight have high

---

Pop Quiz
Do you have Leptin Overload?
Three simple questions uncover your risk

How can you tell if leptin overload is the source of your joint troubles? Well, it's surprisingly simple to find out. Just answer these three questions:

1.) Have you tried other joint support supplements, like glucosamine, with no results?

This is a big red flag, because things like glucosamine don't have any effect on leptin. So if that's the underlying source of your troubles, it makes sense that they wouldn't work. Remember, Leptin Overload could be the reason 4 out of 5 people with stubborn, achy joints CAN'T seem to get relief.

2.) Do you worry about your "numbers"?

I'm talking specifically about these four main health markers: blood pressure, cholesterol, blood sugar, and waistline. If you have trouble keeping them in check, it's a huge signal that your leptin levels could be high.

3.) Do you have trouble losing weight?

Stubborn weight gain is the biggest red flag of all that you could be suffering from Leptin Overload. As I mentioned above, fat cells actually churn out leptin...so the more excess pounds you're carrying around, the more leptin you have in your system. And in your joints.

---

levels of leptin not only in their blood, but also their synovial fluid. And this is particularly true for women.

Synovial fluid is a gel-like substance in your joints. It works like a lubricant, reducing friction in your joints when you move. And a growing number of studies show that the higher the leptin levels in your synovial fluid, the more joint pain you'll have.

The silent symptom of metabolic syndrome

There's also a strong link between leptin and metabolic syndrome—which, as you're well aware, can lead to chronic health concerns. High levels of leptin have been linked to high levels of insulin as well as insulin resistance…along with high blood sugar, high blood pressure, high cholesterol and, of course, weight gain.

In other words, joint pain is another symptom of metabolic syndrome. And it's a symptom that almost no one is looking for.

Here's a recap of what we know…

- The more you weigh, the more leptin you're likely to have circulating in your blood and your joints.

- High levels of leptin have been linked to inflammation, insulin resistance, and increased insulin levels

- High levels of leptin also speed up the progression of arthritis

- All of these factors are associated with metabolic syndrome.

In fact, as many as four out of five people with joint pain also have metabolic syndrome.

Quite a vicious circle, isn't it? Of course, you can help address all of these issues by losing weight. But that takes time. That's why I was so excited to learn about a revolutionary new supplement called OralVisc® that can help you rein in excess leptin WHILE you're losing weight.

The next generation of joint support

OralVisc was developed by the same team of scientists who made one of the most important joint health discoveries in history—the first-ever naturally extracted form of hyaluronic acid, a powerful lubricating compound.

That discovery revolutionized the way we think about "cushioning" the joints…and, truly, changed the supplement world forever. So when I heard they'd uncovered an even bigger breakthrough, I met with them personally to get a firsthand look at their work.

They told me that hyaluronic acid is just one member of a family of nutrients called GAGs (glycosaminoglycans). And they've been tirelessly analyzing different combinations of GAGs in an attempt to find one that could address Leptin Overload.

But every time they changed the combination, they got wildly different results. In fact, one little change could render the whole thing worthless. So they tested and retested for 3 YEARS until finally they hit on the perfect GAG combination—in the exact ratio you need—to conquer Leptin Overload.

They named it OralVisc, and this breakthrough combination is the only nutrient complex that's been clinically tested and shown to defeat Leptin Overload.

Clinical studies show whole-body benefits from OralVisc

Researchers gathered 40 men and women who had had knee pain for at least 10 months. The average age of the participants was 61, and they had an average BMI of 35 (a BMI of 18.5 to 25 is considered normal weight).

The researchers divided the participants into two groups. For three months, one group took 80 mg a day of OralVisc, and one group took a placebo.

At the end of the study, the OralVisc group scored significantly better on joint pain tests. The average pain score of the OralVisc group dropped from 40.3 at the beginning of the study to 27.6 at the end. But the placebo group's score stayed almost the same: from 40.5 to 39.6.

The OralVisc group also had reduced inflammatory markers in their blood and synovial fluid. And they had lower levels of bradykinin, a substance in the joints that starts the inflammation process and stimulates pain receptors.

Even more impressive, the leptin levels in synovial fluid dropped 24 percent in the OralVisc group. But they actually increased 3 percent in the placebo group.

And if that weren't enough, the OralVisc group also had 19 percent lower triglyceride levels than the placebo group.

Can you see why I'm so excited about OralVisc? It's a true breakthrough in joint health. It's the only joint supplement that targets leptin. And based on the research, leptin may very well be the hidden culprit behind aching joints in the vast majority of people. So OralVisc could provide the relief you just haven't been able to get from other natural joint formulas.

Arthritis relief that works just as well as conventional painkillers—without the side effects

Because OralVisc takes a little time to work, I recommend combining it with a fast-action boost. It comes from a soothing, "feel good" plant that's probably in your refrigerator right now—in a bottle of ice-cold beer.

But it's not the alcohol. It's the hops, the plant that gives beer its satisfying "bite."

Hops have a secret talent most people don't know about—and it's not the kind of thing that comes up in conversation at the pub. Hops can help balance one of the most infamous causes of joint inflammation: the COX-2 enzyme.

Keeping COX-2 under control is one of the FASTEST ways to feel better—and it's reassuring to know people have been enjoying hops for more than 12 centuries.

But you can't take any ol' hops. The simple truth is, regular hops have a chemical in them that slows you down and makes you feel sleepy. So it's great for a nightcap, but it's the last thing you want in your joint supplement.

I recommend a unique type of hops called Perluxan®—it has the soothing benefits you need…without the "sandman effect" that can slow you down.

It works so well and so fast, you can begin to feel it in just 2 hours!

And in a clinical study, the active ingredient, Perluxan lowered overall joint discomfort by an astonishing 54 percent.

Study participants who used it for 14 days reported that they could get around more easily. Plus, they could comfortably sit, stand, and lie down without pain getting in the way.

Wipe out crippling leg pain with this step-by-step strategy

I have to admit—peripheral artery disease (PAD) is a tough problem to solve. At the moment, lifestyle changes are usually the best answer that even mainstream medicine has to offer.

Now on one level, this approach represents a refreshing change of pace. But PAD presents some unique challenges that make it difficult to make the changes that can provide the relief you so desperately need.

In a nutshell, PAD restricts the arteries leading to your limbs—blocking nutrient, oxygen, and blood flow. It's not quite the urgent health crisis that coronary artery disease is. (When blood flow is blocked to your heart, you have a heart attack and could die.)

But as you already know, it can erode your quality of life just as quickly.

Leg pain and cramping—a phenomenon called "intermittent claudication"—is the most notorious hallmark of PAD. It can result from even a short stroll around the block. And it can be downright crippling. So it can be pretty frustrating when you're told that you need to move more in order to improve your condition.

This is good advice, of course—I give to patients myself. But I also always offer some additional recommendations that can steer you toward recovery—and get you back on your feet, comfortably.

Of course, a healthy diet—like my New Hamptons Health Miracle, which includes lots of healthy fats and oils from sources like avocado and macadamia nut—is an essential first step.

But with PAD, there are additional factors you need to address too. Most importantly, you want to boost circulation. This means keeping your platelets slippery so they can make it through your blood vessels freely. And in order do that, I recommend a handful of key supplements:

- Pycnogenol—200 mg per day

- Fish oil—3 grams per day of EPA and DHA

- Vitamin E—1,200 IU per day of a full-spectrum product that includes tocotrienols and tocopherols

- Ginkgo biloba—120 mg per day

- Turmeric—250 mg per day

- Citrus bioflavonoids (250 mg of diosmin, 25 mg of hesperidin, and 50 mg of quercetin, in two or three divided doses over the course of the day)

- Magnesium orotate (60 mg per day, depending on your individual needs)

Another solution you might want to try? Chocolate. Yes, really.

As part of a recent study, researchers recruited 20 men and women with PAD. These subjects gave blood samples and then participated in walking challenges over the course of two days.

First, the subjects walked as far as they could on a treadmill, while researchers recorded times and distances. Then the researchers gave the subjects a snack of roughly 1.5 ounces of dark chocolate.

Two hours later, the subjects hopped on the treadmill again. And results showed that they were able to walk for 17 seconds longer and nearly 40 feet farther than they did before.

The subjects also had fewer signs of inflammatory oxidative stress. As well as higher levels of nitric oxide (NO). And as you might recall, NO is essential for relaxing and widening arteries, which, in turn, increases circulation to every part of your body.

So it's no wonder that this "treatment" delivered measurable improvements in PAD patients. Though it's worth noting that the same regimen delivered zero improvements when researchers substituted milk chocolate for polyphenol-rich, 85-percent cocoa dark chocolate.

In other words, a Hershey bar isn't going to do the trick here. You need a high-quality cocoa product to replicate these results.

In combination, all of these strategies should make a huge difference to peripheral circulation—and ultimately, to your comfort and ability to exercise.

And once you start adding regular physical activity into the mix—even if it's just a short 20-minute walk after dinner every evening—there's a good chance you'll be able to sideline PAD symptoms permanently. But as they say, one step at a time.

A perfect, scalpel-free cure for excruciating gallbladder attacks

Gallbladder removal (technically known as cholecystectomy) is actually the most common surgery performed in the United States.

Primarily because most mainstream doctors use it as the go-to prescription for every minor gallbladder flare up. But if you ask me, removing an organ as the first-line treatment for any condition is overkill.

The fact is, you need all of your organs—even the ones the "experts" think are useless. The appendix is a perfect example. Up until about a year ago, no one thought it served much of a purpose in the body. So, like gallbladder removal, appendectomies were viewed as "no big deal."

But we now know the appendix houses all the good bacteria your body needs to stay healthy.

And your gallbladder serves an equally important function.

Your gallbladder is a pear-shaped organ under your liver. It stores bile, a fluid made by your liver to digest fat. Your gallbladder releases bile into the stomach and intestines through a tube called the bile duct.

Most of the time, this system works perfectly, and you never notice your gallbladder. Problems arise when something blocks the flow of bile from the gallbladder through the bile ducts. The primary culprits are usually gallstones. Gallstones are hardened deposits of bile. And if they get lodged in your bile ducts, you'll know it.

Symptoms can be very painful and usually occur after you eat. The most common ones include nausea, vomiting, cramping, or sharp pain in the abdomen, back, or just under the right arm. Attacks usually last anywhere from an hour to four hours.

If you experience these attacks regularly, your doctor will probably tell you that you need surgery. But unless your gallbladder is diseased or actually ruptured, surgery should be your last resort. Especially since there are other things you can try first.

In fact, there's one step I recommend to every person who's ever experienced a gallbladder attack...

Whether you're prone to gallstones or have only had one attack, the first thing I would recommend is to switch to my New Hamptons Health Miracle immediately.

You hear a lot about high-fat foods causing gallbladder attacks. And that's true to some extent. But it's a major oversimplification. I don't know anyone who's had a gallbladder attack after eating a piece of salmon or an avocado. Both of which are considered "high-fat" foods (and both of which are staples on my New Hamptons Health Miracle).

But that's because they're rich in monounsaturated fat. The kind that actually helps promote healing throughout the body. Not the processed, saturated kind (which DOES contribute to gallbladder attacks).

Gallstones are also a sign of inflammation in your system. And one of the primary benefits of my New Hamptons Health Miracle is it helps squelch inflammation everywhere in your body. Including your gallbladder.

Once you've made that switch, I also recommend adding more alkaline foods to your diet. This helps even out your body's pH balance.

If your pH balance is too acidic, it can create excess inflammation. Luckily, alkaline foods are easy to find in the supermarket or your local farmers' market. Cucumbers, broccoli, and almonds are just a few examples. You can find more complete lists of alkaline foods all over the Internet.

If you're in the midst of a gallbladder attack, there are a few natural substances that can help ease the pain. I sometimes recommend willow bark or an enzyme formula called Wobenzym. But it's important to see a doctor first if you're in pain.

And unless the pain is really severe, I usually have my patients ride it out. And work on figuring out what brought it on in the first place. (This is one of the few instances where I would recommend keeping a food diary.) Because, usually, a gallbladder attack can be traced back to a particular food or meal. And, more often than not, it's something that isn't good for you anyway.

Yet another reason the New Hamptons Health Miracle is the perfect remedy for gallbladder problems. Not only will it keep you from potentially dangerous surgery, it will also help you look and feel better overall.

The "tap water cure" for banishing painful kidney stones

Kidney stones are one of the most painful conditions you can get. Unfortunately, they're also very common.

But what exactly is a kidney stone? The "stone" is a hardened mass of calcium crystals that get stuck in the urinary tract. So why do some people seem to get them again and again, while others escape them altogether?

Well, it turns out some people are predisposed to get kidney stones because of a common genetic variation in a gene called claudin-14.

Researchers explain that the claudin-14 gene is a gatekeeper between the kidneys and the bloodstream. When claudin-14 is inactive, as it normally should be, the kidneys' filtration system works fine. Any calcium in the urine is allowed to flow back into the bloodstream.

But some people are born with an overly active claudin-14 gene. So they have an increased risk of kidney stones. But there's an easy way to reduce that risk.

Drink lots of water.

When people don't drink enough, claudin-14 is even more likely to prevent calcium from re-entering the blood. And when calcium builds-up, kidney stones develop.

So how much water do you need? I always recommend drinking the amount of water in ounces that your body weighs in kilograms. Which is easier to figure out than it sounds.

A kilogram is 2.2 pounds. So just divide your weight by 2.2, and that's the number of ounces of water you need every day.

CHAPTER 5

A simple sugar shot soothes pain in up to 90% of patients

I've never been in favor of steroid injections for relief of any type of pain—neck, back, or joints.

Under the best of circumstances, steroids only provide a quick fix and don't do anything to remedy the long-term problem that's causing the pain. At worst, I've seen hundreds of cases of contaminated steroid preparations that have caused fatal fungal brain infections in unsuspecting people.

Fortunately, there are many natural alternatives to steroids for managing pain. And for joint pain specifically, new research shows that manual and physical therapies and another little known natural treatment—prolotherapy—are just as effective as steroid injections. But without any of the risks.

Let's take a look at this natural therapy and the compelling new research that shows how it can end your joint pain—forever.

Prolotherapy is based on the premise that chronic joint pain at least partially results from inadequate repair of connective tissues around the joints. Prolotherapy practitioners inject minute amounts of substances such as cornstarch, sugar, or a cod liver oil mixture into those connective tissues.

The body reacts by promoting tissue repair and growth—like tiny, cellular "micro-sutures" that tighten up the tissues without surgery. Taking vitamin C before and after prolotherapy treatments also helps lay down the collagen that cross-links the new connective tissues to make them strong.

You have to wonder why such a simple, effective, safe, and inexpensive treatment for something as common as joint pain remained hidden for so long. Of course, it probably has something to do with the fact that prolotherapy doesn't require expensive (yet often ineffective) surgery—and repeat surgery—by the burgeoning orthopedic industry.

The good news is, prolotherapy has recently been attracting more interest from researchers. And they are reporting fantastic results. For instance, a new study looked at 38 adults who had at least three months of osteoarthritis-related knee pain. During the first, fifth, and ninth weeks of the study, the participants were given prolotherapy injections containing dextrose (a sugar) in the connective tissues surrounding their knees. More injections were given to those who needed them at 13 and 17 weeks.

The researchers concluded that these prolotherapy treatments resulted in significant levels of safe, sustained improvement in mild to severe knee pain, function, and stiffness. And there were no adverse effects. In addition, at the end of the study, 91 percent of the people who had the prolotherapy treatments said they would recommend them to others with painful knee osteoarthritis.

If you'd like to try prolotherapy yourself, it's much easier today to find a practitioner than it was a decade ago. I offer it myself at my clinic in New York. But there's an entire website, www.getprolo.com, listing practitioners throughout the United States. Considering the proven effectiveness and safety of prolotherapy and physical therapy for joint pain, there is truly no need for you to ever have steroid injections. And, certainly, never consider surgery until you have tried these much safer and more cost-effective alternatives first.

Chapter 6

The silent enemy that's stealing your sleep… and the drug-free prescription that will put your insomnia to bed

It's 3 o'clock in the morning. And yet, you're still awake, pacing the house. *Again.*

And it only gets worse from there. When you do manage to get back to sleep, you're still exhausted when the alarm goes off.

So you pull yourself out of bed in that all-too-familiar fog. You brew a pot of coffee. And you hope it's enough to help drag you through your day, until you finally tumble back into bed, exhausted…

…and completely unable to sleep.

If this vicious cycle sounds familiar, I want you to stop what you're doing and listen. Maybe you've given up on the idea of waking in the morning, refreshed and full of energy. Maybe your doctor diagnosed you with insomnia and handed you a prescription for Ambien, Lunesta, or one of its cousins.

But before you head to the pharmacy out of sheer desperation, hear me out. Those sleeping pills aren't going to fix anything. Because, chances are, insomnia *isn't* really your problem.

The fact is, inability to sleep is just a symptom—not a disease. And in my clinical experience, the underlying cause is a diagnosis conventional medical doctors would *never* make. In fact, I would bet that they've never heard anything about it. And they certainly wouldn't know the first thing about helping you fix it.

But I do. That's why my practice is full of people who get incredible sleep every single night without dangerous drugs. And today, I'm going to tell you how *you* can, too.

How chronic fatigue is keeping you awake

You might think fatigue would lead to sleeping too much. But that couldn't be less true. In fact, "fatigue" is exactly what leads to the inability to get quality sleep.

In my clinical experience, adrenal gland exhaustion is the most common culprit behind insomnia.

And one of the telltale signs of adrenal burnout is trouble sleeping. Particularly waking up around 3 a.m. every night. Why? To answer that question, let's talk again about what adrenal fatigue is, and what it means for your body.

In simple terms, adrenal exhaustion sets in when stress overwhelms these glands' ability to generate key fight-or-flight hormones, like adrenaline and cortisol.

Your body releases these hormones to put you on alert in the face of danger—whether it's a physical threat, illness or injury, a family crisis, or just rush-hour traffic. (It's all the same to your body.)

When your adrenal glands are working properly, they stop releasing these hormones shortly after the perceived danger has passed. But if you're under too much stress for too long, things start to go haywire.

Your cortisol levels stay high. Your body stops "listening" to it properly. And eventually, your adrenal glands "burn out" and stop producing enough stress hormones, even when you need them.

And it's this confused state that's *really* driving your insomnia.

Cortisol in particular plays an important role in managing your body's restorative sleep cycles. When you're healthy, cortisol levels peak around 8 a.m. You hop out of bed ready to start the day—and you don't even reach for the snooze button on your alarm.

On the other hand, cortisol levels should be at their lowest between midnight and 4 a.m.—when most people are sleeping soundly.

If your cortisol levels are high when they shouldn't be, you'll be too wide awake to sleep. But cortisol also plays a role in blood sugar regulation. And if it dips too *low*, it could take your glucose levels with it.

This floods your body with adrenaline. And it wakes you up in a wired, desperate search for emergency fuel—usually in the form of carbs or sugar—right around 3 in the morning.

So those middle-of-the-night fridge raids? Well they actually point to some serious hormone problems. Fix the imbalances, and you won't be waking up starving in the middle of the night any more. In fact, you won't be waking up in the middle of the night at all.

A whole new take on tackling insomnia

In order to get better sleep, you have to get your body's stress response back into balance.

Unfortunately, though, eliminating stress simply isn't enough. When you're dealing with adrenal exhaustion, you need to do more than just *stop* the damage. You need to *repair* it.

And there's not a sleeping pill anywhere that can do that for you.

And as always, it starts with your diet.

When you're slogging through the day, running on fumes, it's tempting to rely on "pick-me-ups" like coffee and candy bars. But these quick fixes are only making your problem worse.

Both coffee and sugary foods crack the whip on your adrenal glands. And remember, you don't want your adrenals to work harder. You want to nurse them back to health. And you can do that by following my New Hamptons Health Miracle.

Protein, vegetables, and healthy fats. Eating this way will keep your blood sugar on track—and help restore balance to your hormone levels. And that will take enormous pressure off of your adrenal glands.

Once you've cleaned up your diet, it's time to take a closer look at your surroundings…

Power off to promote sound sleep

It's a connected world with stimuli everywhere. So your bedroom has to be a safe haven.

Go there when you're ready to sleep. But do everything else in another part of your home. If that's not possible, then at the very least, shut down all your electronic devices 30 minutes before you want to go to sleep, at a minimum.

And yes, that *includes* your Kindle, Nook, iPad, or any other reading tablet.

Recent research from the Mayo Clinic showed that the bright-light diodes that illuminate devices like smartphones, e-readers, and tablets impede secretion of melatonin. And melatonin is the hormone that regulates your sleep-wake cycles.

Needless to say, television comes with the same risks.

So make sure your room is *completely* dark. Power off all electronic devices before you get into bed (or, better yet, keep them out of your bedroom altogether). Anything that may have a light—from your alarm clock to a surge protector—can make a difference in the quality of your sleep. So they should all be turned off.

If you must keep something on (like your alarm clock), at the very least tape a piece of paper over the light to cover it up. Get room-darkening shades for any window that lets in light from streetlamps. And if this still isn't enough, sleep with an eye mask. It may feel strange at first, but you'll get used to it. And it's an adjustment worth making if it helps you get the sleep you need.

Oh, and one more thing. Wear ear plugs. Sound pollution can keep you awake too. And I'm not just talking about sirens or rowdy neighbors. Even if you live in a rural area, the wind, the creaking of the house, the heating/air conditioning, the appliances… all of these things make noise that can keep your adrenal glands in fight-or-flight mode. And that's exactly what you're trying to avoid.

Once you've made the necessary adjustments to your diet and your sleeping environment, there's just one more step left to getting the best sleep you can…

Cutting-edge discovery changing the face of sleep science

You know those tough asparagus stalks you've been tossing in the trash during dinner prep? Turns out, they've been hiding a goldmine all this time.

A cutting-edge enzyme-treated asparagus stem extract named ETAS™ is hitting the market as I write this. And if the research is any indication, it could change the face of stress and sleep management forever.

The secret behind the sleep and relaxation benefits of this new breakthrough is something called heat shock proteins (HSPs). These little molecules are responsible for the soothing, stress-melting effects of a nice, hot bath or an hour in the sauna.

Technically, the release of HSPs can be triggered by several factors, including excess heat and free radicals—which you probably recognize as unhealthy.

But that's the point. HSPs are designed by nature to come to your body's rescue, serving as a protector and repairman for damaged proteins. Proteins are your body's basic building blocks. And HSPs are what allow these proteins to stay functional in the face of the assaults that occur during normal, everyday living.

Your supply isn't exactly limitless, though. In fact, HSP release declines with age. So any strategy that triggers the release of more heat shock proteins is going to do your body some pretty big favors.

But the good news is, you don't need to spend all day soaking in a Jacuzzi or sweating in a sauna to manage this feat. Exercise is one effective way to trigger HSP release. Calorie restriction is another—which explains, at least in part, why these strategies have shown such promising results against aging in studies. But neither of these approaches exactly offer quick results. This is where ETAS comes in…

The "shocking" link between asparagus stalks and a deep night's sleep

The asparagus extract in ETAS is rich in a class of compounds called hydroxymethylfurfural derivatives—and a (much easier to pronounce) molecule called asfural in particular.

All of these compounds trigger the release of a powerful, protective heat shock protein called HSP70. But asfural happens to be particularly good at it. (And as an added bonus, it also has notable antioxidant and circulation-boosting powers.)

In other words, asfural-rich ETAS delivers a heat shock protein windfall directly to your body—along with all the stress-melting, deep-sleep-promoting, anti-aging benefits those HSPs deliver. Except, instead of starving or sweating your way back to total rejuvenation, all you have to do is take a supplement.

Drive down cortisol levels—and send sleepless nights packing

Studies show that ETAS has a significant effect on two major stress hormones: chromogranin A and cortisol. Japanese researchers first confirmed these benefits in the laboratory, where they found that ETAS significantly increased HSP70 expression in human cell lines. Small preliminary studies revealed the same effect in actual human subjects taking ETAS.

Two different clinical intervention trials were published in 2014. The first was a randomized, double-blind, placebo-controlled study of 16 healthy adult male volunteers. (Small, but very well designed.) Results showed that supplementing with ETAS enhanced HSP release compared to placebo.

But that's not all—it also delivered significant improvement to subjects' autonomic nervous system (ANS) parameters. Your ANS is responsible for the physical stress response, such as increased heart rate and respiration.

The second study was also randomized, double-blind, and placebo-controlled—another gold-standard trial. But this time, researchers focused on stress-related hormones and sleep. And just as animal models predicted, ETAS supplementation effectively suppressed cortisol elevation and decreased chromogranin A levels. It also had a significant benefit on subjects' sleep states.

This is just some of the research that's been published in the past two years. And it all tells the same story: That ETAS supplementation can drive down cortisol levels by as much as 80 percent. That it can decrease chromogranin A levels with twice the effectiveness of a placebo. And that it can dramatically improve mental stress, quality of sleep — even mood and energy levels — as a result.

Get your "beauty sleep"… and a whole lot more

Heat shock proteins offer natural repair against protein damage from heat and oxidative stress. Collagen—the compound that gives skin its youthful elasticity—is the most abundant protein in your body. It's also one of the first proteins to succumb to the ravages of time (not to mention UV exposure).

So if you guessed that ETAS doubles as a world-class wrinkle eraser, research suggests you're probably correct. Studies show that heat shock proteins help promote healthy, young-looking skin.

All this, from a humble asparagus extract.

In fact, I'm so impressed by the research on ETAS, I worked with the manufacturer to secure an exclusive supply.

If you struggle with stress and occasional sleeplessness, I encourage you to check it out. Because the sooner you boost your body's natural production of heat shock proteins, the sounder you'll sleep…the more rejuvenated you'll feel…and the healthier you'll be as a result.

ETAS is the most exciting advancement in sleep science I've seen in a long time. But just as there are many causes of sleeplessness, there are several ways to deal with it. Here's a look at a few other sleep-promoting nutrients…

Five supplements to help you sleep like a baby

There are five nutritional supplements in particular I prescribe to sleepless patients, above and beyond my basic adrenal support protocol. And I'll begin with the two supplements that you should *always* take:

- **5-HTP.** This will induce drowsiness at bedtime. But it also works on neurotransmitter levels by raising serotonin and other key chemicals in your brain. This helps to regulate your body's sleep/wake cycle, as well as to support your adrenal glands.

Safe and effective doses range anywhere from 100 mg to 5,000 mg at bedtime. (Though most people don't need more than 1,000 mg.) It's a big range, but start with the smallest dose and work your way up, 100 mg at a time, until you notice a difference in how quickly and easily you're able to drift off to sleep.

If it happens the first night, great! But don't fret if it takes a couple of weeks. 5-HTP is very safe.

- **SAM-e.** This amazing amino acid helps regulate neurotransmitters. And they're just as important as your hormones in the pursuit of deep, restorative sleep and adrenal health. Both are responsible for sending critical messages that regulate your body's biological rhythms. I recommend 400 mg every morning.

Unless you're already taking antidepressant medications, 5-HTP and SAM-e should form the core of your sleep restoring supplement regimen. From there, you can mix and match these next three nutrients to find the combination that delivers the best results for you:

- **L-theanine.** This is the calming agent in green tea. It helps relax your mind so you—and your body—can forget about the troubles of the day. I recommend 200 mg 30 minutes before bedtime and 200 mg in the morning.

- **GABA.** This is a neurotransmitter that helps your brain relax. I recommend 800 mg 30 minutes before bedtime.

- **Melatonin.** I can't overstate the importance of melatonin. Your body generates this hormone not only to help you sleep, but also to shore up your immune system. And not surprisingly, production drops significantly with age.

Melatonin and cortisol also fight each other for dominance. And if your cortisol levels are elevated at night—as they often are in cases of adrenal exhaustion—this could interfere with melatonin's activity. That's why I recommend 3 mg at bedtime to start. But if you need to, you can work your way up to a maximum of 21 mg.

You'll likely need to continue to take these supplements until you get your adrenals back on track, and your energy—and sleep quality—starts to soar again. Then, you can gradually wean yourself off of them when you feel ready.

But remember, like I've mentioned before, it can take as long as a year to reach this point. So don't give up if you're not seeing immediate results.

Because at the end of the day, we're talking about two twin conditions. If you're not sleeping, your adrenals can't repair themselves. And if your adrenals are exhausted, you can bet you won't be getting quality sleep. So addressing one issue always requires addressing the other.

It's a complex problem, no doubt about it. But it doesn't have to be complicated to solve. All you need is a single, comprehensive plan—one that covers enough bases to allow your body to regain its natural balance.

And now, you have one.

Shining a nightlight on burnt out adrenals

Do you suffer from…

- Chronic waking around 3 a.m.?
- Urgent carb cravings—especially late at night?
- Unbearable sleepiness (but difficulty actually sleeping)?
- Clouded thoughts?
- Excessive caffeine use to get through a day? (In other words, more than just a cup or two of coffee in the morning.)

Are you...

- Stressed out from work, children, life?
- Working long hours only to come home and take care of household matters?
- Eating poorly?

If you answered yes to most or all of these questions, guess what? You aren't an insomniac. You have adrenal fatigue, and it's stealing your sleep.

But if you want solid proof, two simple blood tests can deliver it.

First, have your fasting cortisol levels checked. If they're too low (less than 10) or too high (greater than 20), then you may have a problem. And if your fasting DHEA-s levels are off, too, adrenal fatigue is a given.

DHEA-s is another hormone that originates in your adrenal glands. Your level will vary with your age and gender. But generally speaking, they should fall around 400 for men and 300 for women.

My tried-and-true protocol for battling adrenal exhaustion...

There are eight supplements I recommend to all my patients who need strong adrenal support:

DHEA. This is a hormone that will give your adrenal gland a much-needed rest. I recommend anywhere from 5 to 50 mg per day, depending on the case. (But do not take this if you have a hormonally related form of cancer or if you're a pregnant and lactating woman.)

Rhodiola rosea. This is an adaptogenic herb. Which simply means that it can help to steel your body—including your adrenals—against stress. I recommend 30 mg, three times per day.

Schizandra chinensis. This works a lot like *Rhodiola*, and helps to stabilize your adrenal gland. I recommend 60 mg, three times per day.

Ashwagandha extract. This is yet another adaptogen that guards against stress, and enhances immunity. I recommend 150 mg, three times per day.

Eleutherococcus sinensis root extract. Also known as Siberian Ginseng—and another adaptogen. I recommend 150 mg, three times per day.

Panax ginseng. This is also a classic adaptogen. I recommend 50 mg three times per day.

Phosphatidylserene. This is a component of your cell membranes—and helps to heal damage done by stress. I recommend 50 mg, three times per day

Licorice. For detoxification, I recommend 10 mg, three times per day.

Just bear in mind that it could be six months or more before you start to really see a difference. Your adrenals didn't burn out overnight… and they won't recharge overnight either. So stick with the protocol, even if you think it's not working. Because it will pay off in the end.

Popular sleep aid takes on cancer, diabetes, migraines, and more

Sure, a good melatonin supplement can be a lifesaver for an insomniac. But melatonin's benefits go well beyond a good night's sleep.

This hormone originates in your pineal gland. Its release is based on your level of light exposure. During the day, your body generates little to no melatonin. And production peaks after dark, about three to five hours after you go to sleep.

So melatonin plays a key role in regulating your body's natural circadian rhythm (your natural sleep/wake cycle). Which is why melatonin supplements are a popular, all-natural sleep aid.

But here's something you might not have guessed about melatonin: I also use it to boost my patient's immune systems.

Research has revealed melatonin as an anti- inflammatory and antioxidant powerhouse. It soaks up health-robbing free radicals. And it mobilizes key immune cells in your body—including T lymphocytes, monocytes, and your first line of defense, natural killer cells.

So melatonin's other surprising benefit really isn't so surprising at all: It may also help prevent cancer.

Shrinks even the most stubborn tumors— and significantly boosts survival time

Research shows that low levels of melatonin are linked to breast cancer. Lab studies confirm this connection, showing increased cancer cell growth in low melatonin conditions—and slowed cell growth with higher levels.

Clinical studies, meanwhile, show melatonin supplementation may be an important adjunct therapy for women with breast cancer—helping to buffer the body from chemotherapy side effects like platelet depletion. One small study even showed that adding melatonin to tamoxifen treatment resulted in modest tumor shrinkage among 28 percent of breast cancer patients who weren't seeing improvement before.

This same study showed improvement in survival rates among men with metastatic prostate cancer, too—as well as patients with unresponsive uterine cancer and melanoma.

And those are just a couple of highlights. Research points to significant increases in survival time among a variety of solid tumor cancers— including brain and lung cancer—with melatonin treatment.

Of course, immune modulation and cancer prevention are just two major "off-label" uses for melatonin. But there's a lot more where they came from.

Cut your risk of diabetes in half while wiping out migraines for good

Data from the Nurses' Health Study recently showed that high levels of melatonin secretion can cut your risk of type 2 diabetes in half.

Scientists have found melatonin receptors in pancreatic cells. And previous research has pointed to the fact that this hormone could somehow be involved in blood sugar metabolism. So the idea that melatonin could protect against diabetes isn't exactly a stretch.

But there's another strong association here that bears mentioning.

Research has also linked sleep disruption to type 2 diabetes. One study showed that men who get less than five hours of sleep per night are *twice* as likely to end up with diabetes as men who regularly clock at least seven hours.

But this link doesn't just apply to diabetes. Researchers have also connected circadian rhythm disruptions to migraines, too. In fact, another recent trial showed that a 3 mg dose of melatonin was as effective of a 25 mg dose of amitriptyline (a tricyclic antidepressant) when it comes to warding off this debilitating condition.

Even better, melatonin supplementation came with lower rates of daytime sleepiness. And it didn't contribute to weight gain, either. (Both of these are common side effects of amitriptyline.)

In fact, subjects taking melatonin actually *lost* weight.

And that's not all…

An all-natural solution for PMDD, arthritis …even sunburn

Research on the topic isn't extensive, but studies have noted abnormal melatonin secretion in cases of premenstrual dysmorphic disorder (PMDD), too. Women suffering from the condition have shorter duration of melatonin secretion and lower melatonin levels.

One recent pilot study looked at hormone levels and mood changes in two small groups of women— five with PMDD and five age-matched controls—over the course of their menstrual cycles.

Not surprisingly, women with PMDD scored much higher than controls on symptom scales measuring depression, tension, and irritability. And as you would expect, their moods worsened significantly in the days following ovulation.

Meanwhile, researchers found that 24-hour melatonin levels dropped significantly among the PMDD sufferers when they were experiencing symptoms. They also noted big differences in nighttime melatonin levels among the two groups.

In women with PMDD, nocturnal melatonin secretion was much lower—which might explain the insomnia reports that so often accompany this condition. (Sound sleep is melatonin's calling card, after all.)

Ultimately, the study authors proposed that abnormal melatonin secretions contribute to imbalances of serotonin—the body's natural happy chemical—in women with PMDD.

I'm not surprised that serotonin might be a major smoking gun behind PMDD. And that's probably why Prozac (under its new name, Sarafem) is now prescribed for this condition.

But why take risky drugs when you can just take melatonin? Especially since studies also support melatonin's benefits against a number of other conditions—including rheumatoid arthritis and neurodegenerative diseases, like Alzheimer's and Parkinson's.

Some small, preliminary trials suggest it could also help against common conditions like IBS… and even sunburn.

So whether or not you've been struggling with sleeplessness, you might want to consider adding melatonin to your permanent supplement rotation. I recommend a starting dose of 3mg (and never more than 15 mg) at bedtime. Feel free to experiment over time in order to find the dosage that works best for you.

Chapter 7

15 Foods that feed your sexual appetite—
no "little blue pill" required!

For years, I've been telling my patients the same secret I'm about to share with you today: You don't need the little blue pill to rev up your sex life.

In fact, you may not need any pills at all.

There are dozens of easy ways to get the libido boost you crave simply by indulging in some delicious—and decadent—foods. So let's start with one of the more well-known aphrodisiacs and take it from there...

Igniting the spark

The first food that comes to mind when you say the word "aphrodisiac" is the oyster. Raw oysters are the richest source of natural zinc.

Zinc has been shown to increase testosterone production. And testosterone is the hormone that controls sex drive in both men and women.

So, yes, even women need to make sure their testosterone levels are optimal (something many mainstream M.D.s completely overlook).

Of course, I've found that when it comes to oysters, there doesn't seem to be any "in between"—you either love 'em or you hate 'em. But don't worry if you fall into the latter category...I've got lots more ground to cover. And I can guarantee that my list of aphrodisiacs has something for everyone, including some items that might surprise you.

Like black tea, for example.

It has been used by the Chinese for centuries to enhance sexual performance. And there have been a handful of clinical studies to back up that traditional use—including one published a few years ago in the *Journal of Ethnopharmacology*.

In this study, researchers noted that black tea offered "marked aphrodisiac activity." Even better, the effects occurred quickly—and didn't cause any harmful side effects.

And if you want to bump the libido-boosting effects up another notch, throw a few cloves into the cup while you're steeping your tea. Some research published in the journal *BioMed Central* showed that clove may enhance both performance and desire.

Granted, these particular studies were done in mice, which isn't typically my first choice when looking for supporting data. But given their long histories of use—not to mention their spotless track records in terms of safety—there's no reason not to give black tea and clove a try.

Of course, it can't hurt to support the mechanics involved in a healthy sex life while you're at it…

Stoking the fire

Topping the list of foods that help support sexual function on a physical level are things that increase nitric oxide production in the body.

Nitric oxide helps blood vessels relax, which eases blood flow throughout the body. And this isn't only good for helping men achieve erections-it also helps bring blood flow to the clitoris, enhancing sexual stimulation for women as well.

Foods that can give you this boost include:

- Garlic. I know—you spent years avoiding "garlic breath" on dates. But it turns out garlic's active ingredient, allicin, has been proven to pump up nitric oxide, making it a key performance-booster. Also, have you ever tried roasted garlic cloves? It's amazingly simple and so delicious served warm with macadamia nut oil…an absolutely sensual indulgence!

- Walnuts, pistachios, and almonds. According to a study in the International Journal of Impotence Research, walnuts and pistachios are abundant sources of l-arginine, one of the primary building blocks of nitric oxide. And almonds are rich in vitamin E, which can also increase nitric oxide.

- Salmon, mackerel, herring, lake trout, sardines, and albacore tuna are rich in omega 3 fatty acids, which deliver a three-fold increase in nitric oxide production, according to the journal Fertility and Sterility. A daily fish oil supplement can also help get the job done (and is a good idea anyway)…but eating the real thing is much more enjoyable, and will boost your efforts even further.

- Watermelon is high in citrulline, yet another nitric-oxide star. (Plus, watermelon's fructose content is remarkably low, so it's one of the fruits you can indulge in without increasing your waistline—or your diabetes risk.)

The next class of biological wonders that enhance sexual performance and desire are flavonoids. The flavonoids in cherries, red, blue, and purple berries cleanse free radicals from to improved blood flow.

But no discussion of aphrodisiacs is complete without mentioning the next item on my list…

Keeping the embers hot

Of course, chocolate lends itself well to romance as it is, but there's quite a bit of scientific evidence behind it, too.

According to a study published in 2006 in the *Journal of Sexual Medicine*, women who reported eating chocolate on a daily basis had significantly higher scores on the Female Sexual Function Index— particularly when it came to desire—than women who didn't eat chocolate. There's also been a tremendous amount of research linking chocolate to improved blood flow. For example, another study, published in 2009 in the journal *Circulation* found that dark chocolate significantly improved circulation—which, again, is an integral part of arousal in both men and women.

Of course, when you're choosing chocolate, it's important to go for the dark variety—which has shown the most benefits in studies. And the darker the better!

The good news is, these days you don't have to go out of your way to find it. I've seen bars containing as much as 80% cacao in the regular supermarket (the higher the percentage the better).

But your best bet is to buy unsweetened chocolate or cocoa powder and sweeten it yourself with stevia. That way you get all the health benefits of the chocolate and none of the harmful effect of sugar.

Finally, rounding out my list of performance boosting delicacies is my personal favorite—butter. It's rich, creamy, decadent…and when it comes from grass-fed and -finished cows (meaning they've never been fed grains), it's a fantastic source of vitamin K2. This vitamin also helps improve circulation to those ever-important areas of the anatomy. You can find organic grass-fed butter in markets like Whole Foods and Trader Joe's.

Chapter 8

The hidden "wine barrel secret" to curing chronic fatigue...and much more

Are you tired? Not feeling as vibrant as you could? You're not alone. Almost all of my patients say they could use more energy. In fact, fatigue is often their primary complaint.

Chronic fatigue is real, potentially debilitating, and has the capacity to destroy everything from careers to relationships. That's why I'm so happy about a promising development in the fight against fatigue.

I'm talking about a supplement called Robuvit®.

Not only does Robuvit contain ingredients that have been shown in studies to help fight both everyday and chronic fatigue, but it can do so much more.

Studies show Robuvit can improve your mood and reduce your allergy symptoms. And it's a powerful detoxifier that supports your liver and lymphatic system. It can even increase sperm count and restore erectile function.

Bottom line: This supplement has something for everyone. And it's all been clinically documented.

More ways tree bark can improve your health

Robuvit is a patented, all-natural extract from French oak trees. Specifically, it comes from oak trees called Quercus robur, which are grown sustainably in France's Massif Central forests.

These oak trees are standardized to contain at least 20 percent roburins—a type of flavonoid.

Humans have been exposed to roburins for centuries from wine and spirits that matured in oak wood barrels.

Researchers think roburins might actually change the function of ribosomes, our bodies' cellular protein factories. Ribosomes help our cells produce energy. So that's a big reason why Robuvit is so good at fighting fatigue.

Robuvit is manufactured by the same company that brought us Pycnogenol® (and you know how highly I think about that supplement, which also comes from the bark of a tree—the French maritime pine). So of course, that means there's plenty of science to back Robuvit, just as there is with Pycnogenol. In fact, there are already a dozen published studies on Robuvit.

Let's start with the research that shows how effective Robuvit is at reducing fatigue and giving you more energy.

A ray of hope for one of medicine's most baffling conditions

As I said above, if you're tired, you're certainly not alone. The majority of Americans report feeling fatigued, and about 1 million have chronic fatigue syndrome (CFS).

CFS can affect every ethnicity, gender, or socioeconomic group. But women are four times more likely than men to suffer from this debilitating disease.

Unfortunately, mainstream medicine has little to offer for CFS. In fact, most conventional doctors don't even believe CFS exists. If you think you have the disease, they're still likely to consider you a "nut". Even despite the new guidelines established by the Institute of Medicine (IOM), which finally classified CFS as a real disease.

But in the world of complementary medicine, we've always taken this condition seriously. And the list of symptoms is a very familiar one to me and my colleagues. Along with persistent fatigue, primary symptoms include loss of memory or concentration, sore throat, enlarged lymph nodes in the neck or armpits, muscle pain, headache, unsatisfying sleep, and extreme exhaustion.

Many patients may also experience secondary symptoms like brain fog;

difficulty maintaining an upright position; dizziness; balance problems; allergies or sensitivities to foods, odors, chemicals, medications, or noise; irritable bowel; chills and night sweats; visual disturbances (sensitivity to light, blurring, eye pain); and depression, irritability, mood swings, anxiety, or panic attacks.

But Robuvit can help fight this awful disease and all of its complications. And fatigue in general.

Combatting CFS at the cellular level

In one new study of older people without CFS, after just four weeks of taking 300 mg of Robuvit per day, the participants had a 25 percent improvement in general fatigue. They also had less tiredness and tension. And a significant improvement in energy levels and positive mental state—without side effects.

Another study involving 80 people (38 with CFS and 42 controls) showed that CFS symptoms improved after four weeks of taking 300 mg a day of Robuvit. The roburins were found to reduce plasma free radicals and oxidative stress in the study participants. Oxidative stress is associated with CFS, which is one of the main reasons Robuvit is so effective for this disease. That and the fact that it increases bioavailability of antioxidants.

Finally, a 2014 study conducted on 91 people with at least five primary CFS symptoms found that six months of supplementation with Robuvit (200 mg a day) had significant effects on the following symptoms:

- 18 percent less weakness and exhaustion
- 29 percent reduction in short-term memory impairment
- 51 percent reduction in joint pain
- 33 percent fewer headaches
- 38 percent reduction in dizziness
- 40 percent less weight fluctuation

Robuvit for mood swings, allergies, cardiovascular disease, and more

If all Robuvit could do was reduce your fatigue, that would be impressive enough. But this amazing supplement can do so much more. Here's what the science says.

Mood improvements. In the study I just mentioned, researchers gave 91 people who took Robuvit or a placebo a standardized mood questionnaire.

The Robuvit group had significant increases in their scores on "positive" words like active, happy, caring, calm, and loving. And they had significant reductions in "negative" words like gloomy, fed-up, grouchy, sad, or tired.

In fact, the overall mood score of the Robuvit group rose from -6.9 at the beginning of the study to a whopping +4.3 at the end of the study, six months later. But the placebo group's mood only improved from -6.5 to -3.4.

Allergies. In a 2013 study, 16 women took 300 mg of Robuvit daily for three days, and 14 women took a placebo. Then they all got a shot of histamine.

Histamines cause many of the common allergy symptoms, like runny noses and itchy skin. There's some evidence that people with chronic fatigue may have extra sensitivity to histamines, and thus more allergic reactions.

After the women got the histamine shot, the researchers measured the red, itchy bump on the skin that the histamine caused. In the Robuvit group, the size of the bump and red area was substantially smaller than the placebo group. That led researchers to conclude that Robuvit may be effective in fighting histamine-related allergic responses.

Cardiovascular disease. One small study showed that Robuvit reduced homocysteine levels. Elevated levels of this amino acid have been associated with heart disease, stroke, and blood clots.

Liver health and detox. The liver is one of the most important organs in your body. It helps regulate blood sugar, proteins, and fat in the bloodstream and plays a key role in removing toxins from our blood. It also processes nutrients from the food we eat, produces cholesterol and albumin (an important protein), and breaks down alcohol.

That's why it's crucial to take care of your liver. And recent research shows that Robuvit is a key way to do it. Researchers found that Robuvit helps normalize elevated liver enzymes and increase albumin levels, which helps reduce liver injury.

Leg swelling. The lymphatic system removes fluid from tissues and transports white blood cells into the bones. When it's malfunctioning, you can get lymphedema—fluid retention and tissue swelling. This often occurs after surgery when lymph nodes have been removed, and is close to impossible to treat.

But in a recent study, 65 people who took 300 mg of Robuvit daily for eight weeks had 15 percent less swelling in their legs. And the group that took 600 mg of Robuvit had 19 percent less swelling. Both groups also had significant reduction in other symptoms of lymphedema.

What's exciting about this finding is that given enough research, Robuvit could prove to be the answer to diabetic peripheral neuropathy and even restless leg syndrome—both of which have no good treatment options in traditional medicine.

Erectile function and sperm counts. One new study shows that a combination of Pycnogenol, Robuvit, and two amino acids actually restored erectile function to normal in just four weeks. (Take that, little blue pill.) And another study showed that after four weeks of taking the same combo, sperm volume and counts improved.

PART II

SHOCKINGLY SIMPLE CURES FOR TODAY'S BIGGEST KILLERS

CHAPTER 9

TauPro: The revolutionary sleep secret that fights Alzheimer's too

You'd be hard pressed to find a more dangerous drug than sleeping pills. In fact, one recent study linked the popular sleep aid Ambien (and others like it) to a fivefold increase in risk of death.

That means sleeping pills could contribute to 500,000 "excess deaths" per year. And let's not forget that they're ridiculously addictive. How they're still even on the market is beyond me.

But still, insomnia is a real issue, and anyone who has ever suffered from it can understand the desperation that drives people to take risky drugs. That's why I was so thrilled to bring you news of a new cutting-edge supplement called ETAS™ last June (I sometimes refer to ETAS as "Tau-Pro" because of how it works. I'll get into that later).

ETAS is an extract from asparagus stems that have been treated with enzymes. It works by tapping into molecules called heat shock proteins (HSPs).

These molecules are what makes you feel relaxed and soothed after spending time in the heat of a bath or sauna. Your body releases them in response to heat (and other potentially harmful environmental factors) in order to protect and repair damaged proteins.

Unfortunately, the body's supply of HSPs isn't limitless, and your natural stockpile declines as you age. This is where ETAS comes in. It contains compounds that trigger the body to release a powerful form of HSP.

In other words, ETAS boosts the body's supply of HSPs, unleashing the relaxing, sleep-promoting, anti-aging benefits they provide.

Hot off the presses

There have been some impressive studies on ETAS published already, but I've been on the edge of my seat waiting for the results of one large and well-designed study that's been in the works for quite some time. Well that study has finally been published, and it turns out that I had every reason to be hopeful.

The previously published studies—including lab studies and ones in human subjects—showed that ETAS didn't just enhance HSP release, it also helped control the stress response in other ways.

First, it decreased levels of two key stress hormones, chromogranin A and cortisol. And second, it improved the autonomic nervous system's response to stress.

And because stress is a sleep-killer, both of these effects help promote restful, restorative, care-free sleep.

The new study built on this previous research—and took it a step further by investigating how ETAS affects psychological stress when taken for longer periods of time. The double-blind, placebo-controlled study included 25 participants who took 150 mg of ETAS per day for 28 days.

The researchers wanted to verify that ETAS has the effects on the autonomic nervous system seen in previous studies. To do that, they measured how participants reacted to mental stress.

Beyond that, they wanted to determine whether ETAS could cut psychological stress markers like fatigue and poor mood. They measured that with a psychology questionnaire that looks at six different measures of emotional wellbeing.

The results were impressive…and they showed that ETAS appears to squash stress in more ways than originally thought.

After 28 days of taking the supplement, participants reported feeling less tired and "heavy." (If you've ever struggled under the weight of chronic stress and poor sleep, you can probably relate to that description.) ETAS also made it easier for people to get out of bed in the morning, which suggests it improved sleep quality. Again, ETAS is proving to be key to that deep, restorative sleep we all need.

Second, ETAS counteracted the harm stress does to the immune system by bolstering secretory immunoglobulin A (sIgA) levels. SIgA is the body's first line of defense against foreign invaders. It is secreted in all mucosal surfaces, including the mouth, nose, throat, eyes, and digestive system. In other words, the key entry points for viruses, allergens, and bacteria.

Protecting mucosal surfaces is essential for a healthy immune system. But when we're stressed, we stop producing as much sIgA as we need. Which explains why when we're stressed, we seem to catch every bug going around.

But this study showed that ETAS can help keep the immune system operating at peak performance, even when you're under stress.

Not only that, but ETAS helped with the actual performance of those mental tasks as well.

A new revolution in memory loss?

Studies on ETAS have shown it boosts a critical heat shock protein known as HSP-70 by a whopping 300%. Why is HSP-70 so important? Because it can do something that no FDA approved drug on the market can do... naturally.

In scientific studies, HSP-70 has been shown to clear both dangerous amyloid beta plaque as well as Tau plaque from the brain. Which, of course, is why I sometimes refer to it as "Tau-pro".

Tau plaque is fast becoming a prime target in the fight against Alzheimer's disease.

Studies on ETAS are still in the early stages but they show it not only wards off stress but also boosts memory.

Of course, it makes perfect sense that ETAS sharpens memory and mental function. I've told you before that to protect your brain—and your memory—adequate restful sleep is non-negotiable.

It's during the deep stages of sleep that the brain processes newly acquired information and turns it into memories.

All the benefits, none of the risk

So to recap, this singular study showed that ETAS:

- improves feelings of fatigue and "heaviness"
- improves sleep quality
- boosts the immune system
- sharpens brain function

And, perhaps the best part? It does all of this safely. In fact, ETAS has been proven safe time and again—in stark contrast to Big Pharma's sleep aids.

Chapter 10

The Halo Cure:

A cut-poison-and-burn-free solution for defying your diagnosis

---

I often speak out against the barbaric nature of conventional cancer treatment.

It's not that I think everyone should opt out. There's little question that chemotherapy and radiation can "cure" this disease. I simply can't believe that, after all these years, they're *really* the best we've got.

Think about it. We live in a day and age where science fiction fodder like space travel and cloning is actually possible. And yet, when it comes to cancer, patients are still informed that their only viable option is to indiscriminately flood their body with poison.

It's the medical equivalent of burning down the barn to deal with the rats. Effective…but senseless. And this reality is made all the more frustrating by the fact that, presumably, it's the best strategy on offer.

So much of my practice revolves around minimizing the horrible effects that come with modern cancer treatment, while aiming to maximize my patients' results. But truly, I envision a day when the first half of this equation becomes completely unnecessary.

And it looks like that day could be arriving sooner than I thought. A new, groundbreaking treatment has recently come onto the scene. And it's shaping up to change cancer care as we know it.

Stunt deadly tumors without devastating side effects

This technology is called tumor treating fields—or TTF, for short. Also nicknamed the "Halo Cure," this non-invasive medical device consists of insulated electrodes which are attached to your skin in the location of the tumor, like a bandage. These electrodes connect to a small field generator, which you wear continuously in a small backpack.

You remove the device to shower or bathe. But otherwise, you're free to go about your daily life without any interference.

That's because the device doesn't deliver an electrical current to the tissue, as with some other forms of electrotherapy. On the contrary, as the name suggests, a TTF device simply generates an electrical field. Unlike an electrical current (which is a flow of charge), an electrical field is the space around a charged particle.

You won't feel this field. But it's able to influence the behavior of highly charged particles. It just so happens that the proteins responsible for cell division fall into this category. And cancer's most notorious calling card is the speed with which malignant cells reproduce.

Simply put, TTF generates an electric field that paralyzes cancer cells as they attempt to rapidly divide. This essentially scrambles their programming and causes faulty reproduction, resulting in daughter cells that are unable to survive. Or, after enough unsuccessful attempts at division, the cancer cells simply give up and die.

Meanwhile, normal non-dividing cells and healthy tissue—including bone marrow, which is responsible for red and white blood cell production—remain completely unaffected. And so do you.

No nausea. No brain fog. No bone-crushing fatigue.

You might have a mild skin reaction to the electrodes. And in very rare cases, patients could experience headaches, tiredness, or muscle twitching. But even the worst case scenario pales in comparison to the average experience with chemotherapy.

And that, quite frankly, is incredible. Especially when you consider the results this system can deliver.

Early lab research shows that TTF really works

That's really the most vital question here: Just how well does this new

TTF technology work? So let's take a look at what we know so far.

The earliest research on this technology focused on the effects of tumor treating fields on cancer cells *in vitro* (test tube) and in animal models. Experiments used a wide range of human and animal cancer cell lines. These included glioma, glioblastoma, melanoma, lung, breast, prostate, and colon cancers.

This is when TTF's future really cracked open. Results showed *significant* activity in terms of apoptosis (programmed cell death) and arrested tumor growth. In fact, animal models revealed extensive cancer cell destruction in less than a week.

These results carried over in animal models of metastatic cancer. This means that TTF may be able to prevent the spread of cancer as well as stop tumor growth. *In vitro* research also suggests that TTF may pose a crucial threat to tumors that stop responding to chemotherapy agents. (A phenomenon called multi-drug resistance.)

These benefits speak pretty loudly for themselves. But as I'm always saying, research in the lab is only worth so much.

And that's what makes the results of clinical studies on TTF so thrilling.

Fights the most lethal form of brain cancer better than standard chemo

The most compelling clinical support for TTF is in cases of glioblastoma multiforme (GBM). It's the most malignant and aggressive type of brain tumor.

A GBM diagnosis is largely considered a death sentence. The five-year survival rate for patients with GBM is less than 5 percent. Most will survive 15 months on average with standard treatment. Without treatment, the disease could take them in as little as three months.

Just last year, researchers completed Phase III trials of TTF on patients with recurrent GBM. (This means they had received treatment for GBM—in the form of surgery, radiation, and chemotherapy—but the tumors started to grow again.)

Of these subjects, 120 received TTF treatment alone, while 117 received chemotherapy. Median survival rate with TTF was 6.6 months—with chemo it was 6 months.

One-year survival rates were the same between both groups—20 percent. But perhaps most significantly, patients enjoyed a much higher quality of life in the TTF group. Which means tumor treating fields offered *at least* the same survival benefits as standard treatment…but with a fraction of the suffering.

Believe it or not, one member of this study has survived on TTF for more than *six years*.

Clinical trials are currently underway to assess TTF's effectiveness in combination with chemotherapy in newly diagnosed GBM patients. And so far, results look promising.

In-vitro analysis reveals that TTF super-sizes chemotherapy's cancer-fighting abilities. (Findings suggest that it boosts cells' sensitivity to cancer drugs by as much as threefold.)

And results in both animal models and actual human GBM patients reflect this synergistic effect. In fact, a combination of TTF treatment and chemotherapy was able to stop disease progression for nearly three years…with overall survival coming in at 39 months or longer.

In a nutshell, TTF therapy more than *doubled* average survival times in newly diagnosed GBM patients. And these are just the results we've seen with one particularly deadly type of cancer.

Casting a new lifeline to lung and breast cancer patients, too

Published results of early trials on advanced non-small cell lung cancer debuted in September 2013. As part of this research, 42 patients with inoperable, progressing stage IIIB and stage IV lung cancer received daily TTF therapy in combination with standard chemo.

It's worth noting that the five-year survival rate for stage IIIB and stage IV non-small cell lung cancer is less than 10 percent and less than 5 percent, respectively. So we're talking about a disease that's every bit as deadly as GBM.

Results showed that nearly 15 percent of the subjects saw a partial remission of their disease. Almost half maintained a stable disease. Average overall survival was 13.8 months.

Just to put this in perspective for you, the median survival time for stage IV non-small cell lung cancer patients—which comprised just over three-quarters of this subject set—is eight months. So these patients lived almost 75 percent longer than usually predicted, thanks to TTF.

Pilot trials, meanwhile, are underway in patients with advanced breast cancer. And preliminary results have been near miraculous.

The first four patients treated to date have seen their tumors shrink dramatically—by 83 percent, 86 percent, 96 percent, and 100 percent. (That's right—that last patient's tumor actually *disappeared* with TTF treatment.)

Growing availability

TTF is a very new technology. The FDA just recently approved its use in cases of recurrent GBM and is currently in the final stages of approval for non-small cell lung cancer. However, the device is already approved for treatment of newly diagnosed GBM and lung cancer in Europe.

And as we speak, trials are also in the works for cases of ovarian, breast and pancreatic cancer. I expect that list to get a lot longer in the years to come.

For an exhaustive list of treatment centers in the United States please visit www.novottftherapy.com.

As for what the future holds? By the looks of it, the possibilities here are truly limitless. And I'll be watching developments very closely, to say the least. This may be the first you've heard of tumor treating fields. But I'm certain it won't be the last.

Chapter 11

The "Mediterranean Miracle Molecule" that strips cancer cells of their "superpower" and kills them on sight

Maybe you've never heard of apigenin. But if you start following my dietary advice, you'll be consuming a lot of it anyway. And believe me, that's a very good thing.

New research suggests that this common phytochemical is also a powerful anti-cancer agent. And it doesn't just *prevent* cancer, either. It can literally stop cancer cells dead in their tracks.

The flavonoid that strips away cancer's superpowers

Apigenin is a flavonoid—an antioxidant powerhouse in the same class as hesperidin and quercetin. It's not a natural-products industry darling, like resveratrol or EGCG. (Not *yet*, at least.)

But one look at the evidence shows that it's only a matter of time before this compound carves out its own place on the supplement shelves.

Scientists have discovered that apigenin launches an attack against abnormal cells on several different fronts—all of which act in tandem to thwart cancer growth.

One of the most recent studies showed that apigenin is able to undermine cancer cells' ability to cheat death (which they do by tricking your body's natural cell cycles). This is the loophole that allows tumors to grow unchecked. (In fact, researchers have found that cancer cells use sugar to do this...but that's a discussion for another day.)

According to this new study, apigenin restores a normal life cycle to cancer cells by interacting with key proteins that influence RNA. This gives the malignant cells a different set of "instructions" that makes them vulnerable to programmed cell death, when they otherwise wouldn't be.

But it's not the only trick apigenin has up its sleeve.

Cancer cells are able to avoid their natural fate by subverting a protein called p53. This is a tumor suppressor that triggers the death of cells with damaged DNA. Research shows that apigenin is able to activate p53. And this lowers cancer cells' resistance to chemotherapy and improves responses to treatment.

Yet another recent study showed that apigenin also blocks vascular endothelial growth factor (VEGF) This is the same factor that triggers angiogenesis—a technical term for the new blood vessels that tumors grow to feed themselves.

To put it simply, apigenin starves malignant tumors. And this slams the brakes on cancer development and growth.

And now, apigenin's unique cancer-fighting powers are at the center of another recent study—this time focusing on one of the deadliest forms of the disease.

A team of researchers treated human pancreatic cancer cell lines with apigenin, along with another flavonoid called luteolin, extracted from celery and artichoke. And they found that these compounds increased cancer cell death rates from 8.4 percent to 43.8 percent.

Their conclusion? Pretreatment with apigenin might significantly boost the effectiveness of chemotherapy in cases of pancreatic cancer.

The researchers made a point of noting that you likely *wouldn't* be able to eat enough of either vegetable to consume the amounts of flavonoids used in this study. And there's always the question of whether lab results will carry over in a clinical setting.

But their hope—and mine, as well—is that this research will lead to the development of new supplements to aid in the fight against cancer.

As of now, stand-alone apigenin products are scant. (Although other sources, like chamomile extracts, are more common.) I expect that to change in the not-so-distant future, as long as studies like this one keep making headlines.

But until then, you can't go wrong by filling up on dietary sources of apigenin. (Check out the box on the next page.)

Eat yourself away from a dozen different cancers

Numerous studies on a variety of human cell lines show that apigenin can help combat a long list of cancers. These include, but are not limited to: leukemia, lung cancer, colon cancer, ovarian cancer, cervical cancer, endometrial cancer, breast cancer, prostate cancer, skin cancer, thyroid cancer, gastric cancer, and liver cancer.

And I've seen it work first-hand with countless patients—like Ivy Posner.

Ivy was given 6 months to live…21 years ago

When Ivy's oncologist gave her 6 months to live she just wanted to see her children get married… But now, 21 years after her first visit to my clinic, she's seen four *grandchildren* born!

In 1993, Ivy's doctor sat her down and gruffly gave her the dreaded news every woman fears… "It's breast cancer, and it's bad."

By that point it had reached stage 4… Her doctor gave her just 6 months to live and suggested the typical regimen of chemo and radiation.

But after seeing chemo and radiation slowly suck the life out of countless friends, Ivy knew she had to take a different route.

That's when she decided to schedule her first appointment with me.

One of the most important parts of her cancer treatment with me was getting more apigenin-rich foods in her diet.

For the most part, these are all Mediterranean diet staples. So once again, if you follow my nutrition advice, your bases in this department should be well covered.

Ivy will be 81 in February… She now has 2 children, 4 grandchildren and still works every day at her job as a librarian.

And she did it without the slightest bit of radiation or chemotherapy.

Aside from the foods mentioned here, you can also find apigenin in supplement form—although at this point, it's not widely available.

Swanson currently offers a single-ingredient apigenin product derived from grapefruit. But another alternative is to look for chamomile extract that's been standardized for high apigenin content.

Apigenin-rich foods include endive, beans, broccoli, leeks, onions, basil, rosemary, oregano, thyme, tomatoes, and especially chamomile, celery, and parsley—just to name a few abundant sources.

Chapter 12

The Complete Remission Blueprint:
Your personal guide to beating cancer with SP-5

TSP-5 is currently the No. 1 natural cancer treatment used in over 700 clinics and hospitals in Japan. Not only is this treatment as thoroughly researched as ANY pharmaceutical cancer drug, but it actually works better!

SP-5 works on ANY type of cancer…breast, prostate, lung, stomach—even brain.

And, not only is SP-5 the most promising cancer breakthrough in the past 150 years…*it's also the easiest.*

If you or anyone you know has ever faced the mainstream "cut, poison, burn" cancer tactics, please keep reading.

Why this mushroom-based product might be the only cancer "breakthrough" you can count on

I don't generally write books about products. Diet and nutrition, yes… but not specific supplements. There has, however, been one major exception in recent years. It's a product with so much therapeutic promise and compelling research to its name, that I'm all too happy to spread the word about it to as many people as I possibly can.

SP-5 therapy involves a mushroom-based immune supplement known in scientific circles as Active Hexose Correlated Compound (AHCC). AHCC works by boosting cancer-killing T-cells in the body to unprecedented levels.

Debates over whether nutritional supplements are an effective (or even safe) way to fight cancer constantly hog health headlines. And in a lot of cases, the controversy is understandable. Published studies deliver conflicting research all the time.

One day, a supplement lowers your risk of cancer. The next day, it raises it. Self-interested research sponsors and inconsistent study methods are common. And that's why we'll probably never get a straight answer where most complementary approaches to cancer are concerned.

That said, I will tell you that my commitment to telling the world about AHCC stems from one simple fact. Unlike some of the other "breakthroughs" you might have read about before, this one actually works.

Why your average medicinal mushrooms aren't good enough

As I mentioned above, AHCC is a medicinal mushroom extract with origins in Japan, where over 700 hospitals use it. Its introduction stateside has been more recent—in the last 20 years or so.

But in that time, reputable universities across the country have subjected AHCC to an expansive body of clinical study.

Needless to say, this is one supplement that enjoys a ton of well-documented research.

Technically, AHCC is a functional food—and it's certainly as safe as a plate of mushrooms. But that's where the similarities end. Edible offerings and most other mushroom-based supplements provide only the fungi's "fruiting body." AHCC, however, draws from the mycelia (or roots) specially cultivated medicinal mushrooms, where active ingredients concentrate.

The manufacturing process breaks down these beneficial components to make them more absorbable. What you end up with is a pharmaceutical-quality supplement packed with immune-stimulating polysaccharides.

Most common mushroom-based health foods and supplements derive their effects from a particular kind of polysaccharide called beta-glucan. The problem is, our bodies don't contain enzymes to digest beta-glucan effectively. So while these other mushroom-based therapies do help somewhat, you're not getting their full potential.

AHCC does contain beta-glucan. But it also contains another type of polysaccharide, called alpha-glucan—or Alpha G. And Alpha G is what sets AHCC apart from other mushroom products. Our bodies are able to break down Alpha G with the naturally produced enzyme amylase. Which means you're getting its full immune-boosting benefits.

But what does any of this have to do with fighting cancer? To answer that question, it helps to take a closer look at the role your immune system plays in both prevention and remission.

The "cure" for cancer starts with your immune system

You have cancer forming in your body every single day...at this very moment, in fact. This is a reality of the disease-forming process that few people realize.

That's because if your body is healthy, you won't even know it's happening. Microscopic tumors develop, and your immune cells hunt them down like Pac-Man to gobble them up before they can grow larger. This is called cell-mediated immunity—and it's sustained by your body's natural killer (NK) cells, macrophages, T-cells, and cytokines.

In fact, doctors assess these immune cell populations in order to form cancer prognoses. Because your odds against any disease are only as good as your defenses.

Ultimately, it's easy to see why having a healthy immune system is so essential. It is, quite literally, a matter of life and death. And as you may have guessed, this immune defense is precisely where AHCC comes into play.

But first, here's what it doesn't do. AHCC doesn't "cure" cancer—at least, not in the conventional sense of the word.

AHCC doesn't attack tumors directly, the way that chemotherapy, radiation, or other conventional therapies do. On the contrary, AHCC heightens this cell-mediated immunity. In other words, it helps your body to launch its own natural defenses...and in doing so, to heal itself.

To that end, AHCC doesn't merely "boost" your immune system. It modulates and directs it, making it smarter and more efficient. The result is powerful support against disease—without the damaging side effects that are hallmarks of modern cancer therapy.

Real research, real patients, real results

AHCC has the benefit of a wide spectrum of research on its side. More importantly, it's solid, reliable research.

Too often, supplement manufacturers cite animal studies as "proof" of their product's effectiveness. This is especially frustrating in the face of cancer prevention claims, because we rarely have assurance that any given compound will work the same in humans, under real world circumstances.

What's more, you'll often see these same studies come from single researchers, without any independent verification. This is not the case with AHCC. My enthusiasm for this product springs in part from the fact that it has been the subject of multiple peer-reviewed and published clinical studies, with multiple authors, examining hundreds of real human patients.

In other words, it's science your doctor can use. And science you can trust.

The body of research on AHCC's anti-cancer properties is vast enough that I couldn't possibly detail all of it here. But what I can offer is a brief overview of some of the most compelling evidence out there—a snapshot of AHCC's "superpowers," if you will.

Higher remission rates...with virtually no risk

Japanese researchers collaborated with scientists at Harvard and Yale to carry out clinical trials here in the United States. And the results have been promising to say the least.

Smaller Phase I trials revealed that even at high doses, AHCC is non-toxic, only causing mild, temporary stomach discomfort and headache in a small portion of subjects. Meanwhile, larger Phase II trials confirmed that AHCC can help to prevent cancer in elderly people by increasing key immune cytokines. These positive effects were noticeable within just four weeks of use, and persisted for at least a month after daily recommended doses ended.

Studies have also shown dramatic increases in survival rates among cancer patients, even those with late-stage or terminal diagnoses. One placebo-controlled study of advanced-stage liver cancer patients, for example, showed that 6 grams of AHCC per day doubled survival time. Other, long-term, placebo-controlled studies reaffirm these results, revealing significantly higher survival rates among liver cancer patients taking 3 to 6 grams of AHCC per day.

These results bear out in a wide range of other types of cancer, as well. A large study of terminal patients with gastric cancer, colon cancer, liver cell cancer, pancreatic cancer, lung cancer, breast cancer, and ovarian cancer showed marked increases in immune cell activity.

But that's not the most remarkable part. Out of 195 patients, this study reported 114 cases of partial improvement or complete recovery. There were also 27 cases in which cancer progression was stopped within 6 months of AHCC supplementation.

These results are stunning, to say the least. And they're just a small sampling of what's out there.

Taking conventional cancer treatment to the next level

It's important to note that AHCC works just as well in conjunction with conventional cancer therapies. In fact, it's a critical complement to popular mainstream protocols.

Using AHCC in combination with chemotherapy can reduce a long list of its most notorious side effects. (This includes nausea, vomiting, appetite loss, hair loss, liver damage, low white blood cell counts, and anemia.) And the fact that research shows AHCC can actually increase chemotherapy's cancer-destroying activity at the same time only adds to its incredible merit.

It's impossible to overstate AHCC's benefits to your health. This supplement has so many perks that go beyond the scope of this report—with studies supporting its use against everything from diabetes and viral infections to chronic inflammation and stress reduction. Enough, in fact, that I've dedicated an entire book to the subject (*The Science of AHCC: Japan's Medical Breakthrough in Immunotherapy* which you can find on Amazon. com). So you can bet I'll revisit this topic again in the future.

But for now, I hope that I've at least left you with a clear idea of why AHCC stands apart from the pack. I like to think that one day, mainstream medicine will give it the widespread recognition it deserves.

Until then, and probably long after, I'll remain one of its most vocal advocates.

Probiotics: A new frontier in the natural treatment of cancer

Immunotherapy is one of the hottest new areas of cancer treatment. It's all about using your body's own immune system to shrink and destroy deadly cancerous tumors. And when you consider that 70 percent of your body's immune system is located in your gut… it's easy to see why many oncologists are starting to look at probiotics as a potent new tool in the fight against cancer.

One of the most interesting ways probiotics are starting to gain attention is as a defense against the devastating side-effects of mainstream cancer therapies such as chemo and radiation. Now, I always recommend a natural approach but I realize treating cancer is a very personal decision and many people are going to go with the most well-known treatments available. And there are cases where these options may be your best (or unfortunately) only choice. In those situations, I always recommend supplementing with a natural option like AHCC (see chapter 6) and now probiotics.

Protecting the body against chemotherapy's harmful effects in order to outlive cancer

Chemotherapy is a tremendous killer of cancer cells but it does so indiscriminately, leaving a trail of millions upon millions of dead healthy

How to put AHCC to work for you

The proper AHCC dosage depends on your specific goals.

As a form of prevention, you'll want to take 1,000 mg of AHCC per day, split into two doses. (I suggest a 500 mg dose in the morning and another at night.) This dosage maximizes general health and strengthens your immune system.

For therapeutic use or as a complementary treatment, I recommend you start with 3 grams of AHCC per day, split into three doses. (That's 1,000 mg in the morning, 1,000 mg in the afternoon, and 1,000 mg at night.) Take this dose for three weeks.

After that, continue to take 1,000 mg daily. (Again, I usually suggest one 500 mg dose in the morning and one at night.)

Starting with a higher "loading dose" initially will increase your NK cell activity at a faster rate, which you can then easily maintain at a lower dose for maximum clinical benefit.

Where to find AHCC

AHCC can be found through various online retailers and in some specialty health food stores. It's also available in a product called ImmPower™ — AHCC from The Harmony Company.

cells in its wake. That's why cancer treatment many times boils down to surviving this assault on the body long enough to let the chemo kill its intended target. It's a race for survival between your body and the cancer inside it. And all too often, the body comes out on the losing end of this medical marathon.

But what if you could find a way to protect your healthy cells in order to endure longer and higher doses of chemotherapy? Doses strong enough to wipe out even late stage cancers and multiple tumors? That's the potential probiotics are starting to reveal to oncologists across the country.

It all started at the University of Michigan where researchers theorized that chemotherapies slow erosion of gastrointestinal tract specifically, resulted in fewer and fewer vital nutrients reaching the body over time and eventually leading to death. They theorized if they could somehow protect the gastrointestinal tract from this devastation, the body could continue to receive life-giving nutrients long enough to outlive the strong doses of chemotherapy needed to eradicate late-stage cancer.

The University of Michigan study that's pointing the way towards a new era of natural cancer treatment

In order to accomplish their goal, the researchers focused on a natural molecule found in the intestines known as R-spondin1. This chemical works to repair any damage done to the intestinal track in order to keep digestion running smoothly and nutrients flowing to the body. The problem with cancer treatment is that chemotherapy destroys intestinal cells at such a rapid rate that the natural amounts of R-spondin1 found in the gut can't keep up with up with the damage. So the University of Michigan team theorized that upping the amount of R-spondin1 in the intestines could potentially protect the intestinal walls long enough to survive large doses of chemo.

To test this theory, university researchers injected a group of mice with R-spondin1 to see how they would fair against lethal doses of chemotherapy. To their surprise, up to **75 percent of the mice injected with R-spondin1 survived** doses of chemotherapy that, pound for pound, would kill most adult human beings. Meanwhile, 100 percent of mice not injected with R-spondin1 died from the chemotherapy.

Triggering your body's own "molecular chemo-shield"

Now this study is only the first step in what could be a decades-long journey for R-spondin1 treatment. But as I mentioned before, R-spondin1 is a completely natural chemical found in all of our intestines. That's why I recommend anyone going through chemotherapy (as well as my healthy patients) take probiotics. This will help ensure natural levels of R-spondin1 and all healthy gut bacteria are replenished on a regular basis.

Just be sure to use one with multiple strains of beneficial bacteria. There are hundreds of strains of probiotic bacteria.

And while research on individual strains continues to build, I believe it's best to support the overall balance of your gut microbiome by supplementing with more than just one strain.

But current research on probiotics doesn't stop with simply protecting your body from mainstream methods of cancer therapy.

New studies are also emerging showing probiotics have the power to help kill cancer outright!

Three specific probiotic strains that are leading the charge in the fight against cancer

There are over 500 different probiotic strains of bacteria in the human intestines but there are three specifically that are starting to pop up in preliminary cancer studies.

One recent study showed that yogurts rich in lactic acid probiotic bacteria were able to slow the growth of colon cancer cells. While milk fermented in the *Lactobacillus helveticus* probiotic strain (commonly found in Swiss and cheddar cheeses) was even able to slow the growth of breast cancer cells.

And even more impressive, a 2007 study found that the probiotic strain *Lactobacillus Casei* (commonly found in cheddar cheese and Sicilian green olives) was able to prevent recurrence of bladder cancer in 74 percent of patients treated!

So while studies are still preliminary and ongoing, if your main goal is to supplement your cancer treatment, I recommend getting healthy amounts of dairy, preferably from hard cheeses such as cheddar and Swiss.

Unfortunately most yogurts also contain too much sugar, which is why I also recommend supplementing with a probiotic with multiple strains of beneficial bacteria.

My three-step plan to ensure you're taking the highest-quality, most effective probiotic

A shocking study revealed most probiotics don't contain what the label says they do. Researchers tested 16 probiotic products available in stores in California and online. And the results were troubling, to put it mildly: Only one of these 16 products exactly matched the contents claimed on the product's label.

The scientists used a DNA-based model to identify the species of detectable bifidobacteria (a type of probiotic) in each of the products. In addition to finding only one product containing the amount and strain of bifidobacteria the label said it did, the researchers also found pill-to-pill and lot-to-lot variations.

One product didn't contain any of the probiotic strains listed on the label. And some products contained strains that weren't mentioned anywhere on the labels.

The easy way to find a quality probiotic

So what's a consumer to do? Here's my three-step plan to ensure you're taking the highest-quality, most effective probiotics.

1. Bigger is not better. A lot of probiotic products you see in pharmacies, health food stores, and vitamin shops try to wow you with the number of colony forming units (CFUs) they deliver. But billions of CFUs are not good for you. In fact, ingesting too many of any one type of bacteria can trigger an autoimmune response and cause complete havoc in your body.

2. The most important thing is getting the right bacteria—and not too many of the same kind. That's why you should look for products with multiple strains of probiotics. With trillions of different types of bacteria cells in your body, a supplement that only has a single strain (or even just a few) won't be much help.

3. Don't forget prebiotics. These are basically "food" for probiotics. Prebiotics make probiotics more effective and longer lasting.

Keep this checklist in mind when you're shopping for a probiotic. (The product label should include all of this information.) Of course, if you want to save yourself the time, you can always opt for the probiotic formula I recommend: Dr. Ohhira's.

Dr. Ohhira's uses special composting and fermentation processes to deliver 12 different strains of live bacteria. Plus, they offer one of the few probiotic products that also contains prebiotics. And Dr. Ohhira's probiotics even include lactic acid bacteria and bacteriocins, which work to kill off the bad bugs while replenishing the good ones. Their formula is also backed by 25 years of university-based research.

Introducing a brand-new probiotic breakthrough: ME-3

Dr. Ohhira's also produces a specific strain of probiotic called lactobacillus fermentum ME-3. It's designed to be taken with a probiotic product like the one I recommended above. Why? Because ME-3 actually does double duty in your gut.

First, it's an excellent antimicrobial that can effectively kill off pathogens and other harmful bacteria that enter the gut. And second, it helps boost your body's production of glutathione.

Glutathione is such a powerful antioxidant that scientists call it the "Master Antioxidant." It's used by every cell in your body—particularly the cells in your liver, cardiovascular system, and immune system. These cells get a lot of daily wear and tear and require extensive antioxidant support.

Unlike other antioxidants, your body can't properly absorb glutathione if it's taken orally, so it had to be given intravenously. But recently, researchers discovered ME-3 actually synthesizes glutathione naturally in your gut. Which means there's finally an easy way to boost your glutathione—simply by taking ME-3.

ME-3 has only been available in the U.S. for a short time, so you're one of the first to know.

Chapter 13

The Master Plan:
How you can beat cancer with curcumin

There's a dirty little secret about cancer that Big Pharma doesn't want you to know. In fact, they make $100 billion every year simply because you don't know this!

Contrary to what you've been led to believe, chemotherapy and radiation cannot cure most people suffering from cancer.

There's a very good reason why—and it's not some big mystery researchers haven't been able to solve yet.

Hundreds of scientists around the world know about it. Nearly 1,000 scientific papers have been published about it.

So why are you being kept in the dark?

Meet cancer's "master cells":
The reason modern treatments FAIL to cure cancer

In the heart of every tumor, you'll find a type of cancer cell nobody wants to talk about—because they are extremely difficult to kill. The truth is, chemo and radiation can't wipe out this type of cell. Many scientists now believe these hard-to-kill cells are the reason that many cancers come back, even after rounds of grueling treatment.

And as difficult as they are to destroy…they are also easily overlooked. PET scans, CT scans, and MRIs can all fail to detect them.

They are called cancer stem cells (CSCs). Usually, stem cells are a good thing in the medical world. You likely associate them with healing and regeneration. But it's a different story with cancer stem cells.

You can think of them like "master cells," because they determine what the rest of the tumor cells do. These lethal cells are in control of how fast cancer grows, where it spreads, and exactly how it manages to evolve and resist treatment time and time again.

In fact, in a mouse study, stem cell researchers discovered that as few as 100 CSCs can cause a tumor to grow right back—while tens of thousands of other cancerous cells cannot.

More malignant, more evolved, and much harder to wipe out

CSCs make up as little as 1% of a tumor's mass. The problem is, conventional treatments like chemo and radiation target the OTHER 99%. These treatments were designed before scientists ever heard of CSCs, and they work by targeting and killing rapidly dividing cells. Trouble is, CSCs divide slowly…which means they can skate through round after round of toxic chemotherapy and intense radiation.

And what happens when a CSC does drink in some of the toxic chemotherapy drugs? Researchers discovered CSCs have a built-in defense mechanism for that—they can pump the drug right back out of the cell.

But that's not the worst part. Chemo and radiation actually make CSCs stronger—32 TIMES STRONGER, according to a shocking UCLA study on breast cancer radiation.

The evidence is strong: If you want to beat cancer, you must defeat CSCs

You can bet Big Pharma knows about this. CSCs were first identified in leukemia back in 1994. Then in 2003, University of Michigan researchers found CSCs in breast cancer. Since then, CSCs have been found in just about every type of solid tumor on the planet.

So the fact that the average cancer patient doesn't know about CSCs—and is never told that chemo and radiation CAN'T kill these cells—is a horrifying betrayal.

Luckily, researchers at 25 universities around the world have come through for you with a groundbreaking discovery…

A natural medical miracle that can destroy Cancer Stem Cells

I'm talking about a powerful, potent compound nicknamed CL-4. It comes from the plant *Curcuma Longa*, and it's been shown to fight cancer at every stage—from early "stage 0" to aggressive, worst-case-scenario stage 4.

You may know this healing substance as curcumin.

Researchers at Baylor University and MD Anderson Cancer Center have led the way in studying curcumin's anti-cancer activity. But the compound has also been studied by elite research teams at Stanford, UCLA, the University of Michigan, the University of North Carolina at Chapel Hill, Purdue University, and many others.

Sixty-three human clinical trials involving curcumin have been completed to date, and five more are underway right now—including one at the Mayo Clinic.

All the evidence we have so far suggests curcumin can outperform chemo—sometimes alone, and sometimes in combination—giving you the best chance of enjoying a cancer-free life. Rigorous studies show curcumin can defeat almost every kind of cancer cell…

- Breast cancer
- Ovarian cancer
- Cervical cancer
- Prostate cancer
- Lung cancer
- Colon cancer
- Stomach cancer
- Bladder cancer
- Brain cancer
- Head and neck cancers
- Myeloma
- Leukemia
- Lymphoma
- Melanoma

This list is impressive. But let's take a closer look at what curcumin can do to destroy CSCs in particular...

Curcumin shuts down 195 cancer-causing signals... while many chemo drugs target just one

With curcumin, Cancer Stem Cells may have finally met their match.

Unlike radiation, curcumin can actually de-program CSCs to act like "regular" tumor cells—which are much easier to destroy with traditional or natural methods.

And unlike many chemotherapy drugs, which target one piece of the cancer puzzle at a time, curcumin has the power to shut down CSCs from 195 different angles.

It's like blowing up every satellite and cell tower in a CSC's communication network. When the cells can't communicate, they can't metastasize.

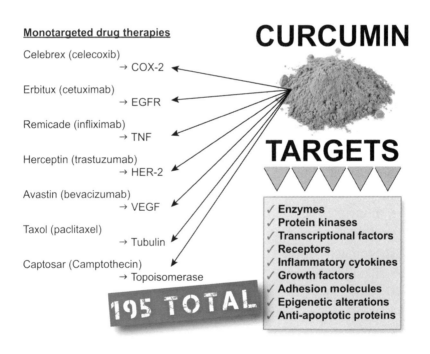

And that's just what researchers have catalogued so far. Dr. Ajay Goel, a colon cancer expert and leading curcumin researcher at Baylor University, believes curcumin has the potential to block thousands of cellular signals.

(And that's exactly why curcumin has been studied as a potential cure for nearly every major health epidemic we're facing today.)

Numerous studies have shown that because of its ability to shut down these pathways, curcumin can:

- Trigger CSC death (apoptosis)

- Stop CSCs from metastasizing

- Prevent existing tumors from progressing

- Make chemotherapy more effective—even when cancer has already become resistant to treatment

Read this before you or someone you love needs chemo…

A growing pile of research shows curcumin makes chemo more effective—so you need LESS of it…and have a GREATER chance of living cancer-free for life.

In fact, a team of stem cell researchers discovered that combining curcumin and the chemo drug cisplatin KILLS 8 TIMES MORE CSCs than chemo alone!

Researchers discovered this in an in vitro study with lung cancer stem cells. In testing, 94% of the CSCs were found to survive a single exposure to low-dose cisplatin. By combining the drug with curcumin, only half survived. The other half were destroyed with just this one dose.

So far, curcumin has been found to supercharge the effects of 12 chemo drugs—including the colon cancer drug 5-fluorouracil (5-FU), which is so well-known for failure that patients call it "5 Feet Under." A study published in the journal *Carcinogenesis* revealed curcumin reduced chemo-resistance to 5FU by 30%.

And that's just the beginning.

- In a Phase I clinical trial of 25 people, curcumin was shown to prevent high-risk precancerous lesions from progressing into cancer. During the study period, 7 people saw their condition improve in 12 weeks.

- In a very small study of patients with advanced pancreatic cancer—one of the most deadly types of cancer known to man—the median survival rate with curcumin was 5.4 months. The one-year survival rate was 19%. By comparison, the median survival for untreated advanced pancreatic cancer is about 3 1/2 months—and with treatment, the median survival rate increases to about 6 months. Animal studies suggest curcumin can increase the effectiveness of chemotherapy and reduce its toxic effects.

- At a U.K. hospital, curcumin was tested as a desperate, last-ditch attempt to save patients suffering from stage 4 colorectal cancer. For 5 out of 15 terminally ill patients, curcumin stopped cancer in its tracks for three to four months. That's more than 200% longer than some chemotherapy drugs—and without the same gut-wrenching side effects.

- A small study tested a curcumin-quercetin combination with a group of patients who had a disorder known as FAP. These patients were at a high risk for colon cancer, currently had anywhere from 5 to 45 polyps, and had previously had part of their colons surgically removed. Three to nine months of treatment with the curcumin-quercetin combo reduced the number of polyps by 60%, and reduced polyp size by 50%.

- Curcumin could offer hope to people suffering from the most difficult to treat form of breast cancer known as "triple-negative." This type of cancer does not respond to any traditional treatments. But researchers in China found that curcumin kills these breast cancer cells, and a team in

Taiwan has had success with combining doxorubicin and curcumin in in vitro studies.

- In animal studies and in vitro testing, curcumin reduced the amount of prostate-specific antigen (PSA) produced by prostate cancer cells, and triggers cancer cell death. In a double-blind, placebo-controlled human study, researchers found that combining curcumin with soy isoflavones suppressed PSA production. At the start of the study, all 85 men had elevated PSA levels and had a prostate biopsy that tested negative for prostate cancer.

Curcumin activates your "Guardian" gene to prevent cancer

Curcumin is also a powerful anti-cancer ally because it blocks the formation of new tumors—to prevent cancer or stop it from coming back.

Normal, healthy cells have a built-in "expiration date." But cancer cells don't. They keep regenerating until a tumor-fighting gene sends them a signal to stop.

When cancer starts to grow, it means your tumor-fighting genes are asleep at the wheel…that is, curcumin bursts in with a bullhorn to wake them up. Once these genes snap back to attention, they force cancer cells to die—slamming the brakes on tumor growth.

Scientists nicknamed one of these genes as "The Guardian" because it helps protect you from nearly every type of cancer. In a groundbreaking human clinical trial from China, with 126 patients, researchers found that curcumin "wakes up" The Guardian and makes it stronger.

In this chart, you can clearly see just how much stronger, by comparing the results to the placebo group:

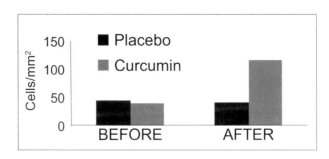

Curcumin triggered the death of more cancer cells. At the same time, the compound helped patients fight a deadly syndrome called cachexia—a form of muscle wasting and weight loss that can be fatal to cancer patients. Weight gain could be seen within 10 days of beginning curcumin.

No pharmaceutical drug on the planet can do what curcumin can do

Many of my patients ask me what the difference is between curcumin and turmeric. Turmeric is the common name of the plant *Curcuma longa*. Curcumin is the active compound within the plant that's used for its medicinal properties.

If you're in a fight for your life, you need to know that not just any old curcumin will do. And while I believe that adding it to your food is beneficial to your health, simply cooking with it is not the best way to maximize its anti-cancer benefits. When turmeric powder is used as a spice, it typically contains only about 3% curcumin.

Early studies uncovered the fact that curcumin is not easily absorbed on its own. (Scientists call that poor bioavailability.) In some studies, patients were given as much as 8 grams (8,000 mg) of curcumin, which can irritate the gastrointestinal system. It is not known how the results could have been affected by using a form of curcumin that was able to be absorbed more easily.

Luckily, nutraceutical technology has come a long way. Now, there are several potent, bioavailable forms of curcumin on the market, including:

- **Meriva®**, a patented time-release curcumin extract. It is a "phytosome" form of curcumin that's paired with fat—a combination that's much easier to absorb. One 2011 study suggests Meriva is absorbed 29 times better than plain old curcumin. In an in vitro study, Meriva was shown to overcome chemo-resistance in colon cancer cells, making the chemo drug oxaliplatin more effective.

- **Curcumin C3 Complex®**, another high-absorption

form of the nutrient that uses nanoparticles. It is currently being used in several clinical trials at MD Anderson Cancer Center, and in a study in Britain on inoperable colon cancer in combination with a chemo regimen known as FOLFOX.

• **BCM-95®**, a bioavailable form that also includes components of turmeric oil. Studies by the manufacturer show that it can be detected in the bloodstream within 1 hour and sustain active levels for more than 8 hours. One study suggests BCM-95 is 6.9-times more bioavailable than regular curcumin. It was used in studies of colorectal cancer to overcome chemo-resistance, and tested in combination with other nutrients against prostate and bladder cancers.

• **Theracurmin®**, a "nano" formulated, water-dispersible extract. It has been studied alone and in combination with chemotherapy for pancreatic, bladder, and prostate cancer, among others. A study by the manufacturer suggests it is 27 times more absorbable than regular curcumin.

These forms of curcumin are "branded," quality-controlled extracts. In general, I prefer these kinds of nutrients because I find they have more science behind them, and they are designed to increase absorption.

Because the research on curcumin and cancer is still emerging, talk to your doctor about the best way to use this powerful extract in your specific treatment plan.

As a general guideline, 500 mg of a bioavailable curcumin extract is a great place to start for overall health and cancer prevention. But the therapeutic doses during active cancer treatment will be higher. Some research suggests 1,000 to 3,000 mg (1 to 3 grams) daily in divided doses, depending on the disease stage.

There are thousands of studies on curcumin in the National Institutes' of Health research database called PubMed. I've cited some of the most interesting studies in the references section of this book. Talk to your doctor about what these studies may mean for your particular case.

Chapter 14

Top Secret Triple-Threat Cure:
How you can wipe out the hidden epidemic
of the Baby Boomer generation

The real culprit behind today's deadliest threats actually goes much, much deeper than you may realize. That's right…there's one sinister syndrome behind things like…

- High blood pressure
- Elevated cholesterol
- Problem blood sugar
- Bone loss
- Sexual dysfunction
- Memory loss
- Vision loss
- Gum problems
- Peripheral neuropathy
- And more

But now, you can eliminate them ALL in ONE FELL SWOOP. With the three affordable, readily available nutrients you'll ONLY learn about right here.

Surprising signs you might be at risk
of this hidden epidemic

While everyone focuses all their attention on the major diseases of aging and how to address each one alone…there's a hidden link lying beneath most of them that could make tackling them ALL easier than ever.

I'm talking about small blood vessel and capillary disease—or impaired microcirculation. And this little-known hazard can lead to some enormous health problems.

In fact, the leading causes of death in this country are almost all related to blood vessels, whether it's stroke, heart disease, or any of the others.

It's all about maintaining healthy blood vessels

Luckily, scientists are starting to unravel the mysteries of this chronic, debilitating (and stealth) illness. And, as it turns out, research is showing that focusing on maintaining—and repairing—your microcirculatory system, or your small blood vessels and capillaries, may be the first step in reversing some of the most devastating complications of today's major diseases.

Unfortunately, that's just not something many people are equipped to do these days. Especially considering that conventional medicine only treats the symptoms of ailing blood vessels (with potentially dangerous prescription drugs to boot). If they recognize the problem at all, that is.

Today, we're going to change all that.

I'm going to give you a complete rundown of all the tools you need to keep your microcirculatory system strong and healthy for the long haul.

But before we get to that, there are...

Three important facts you need to know about this hidden danger

No. 1: When small blood vessel disease occurs, the blood flow to critical areas of your body becomes impaired. Without adequate blood flow, there's not enough oxygen being delivered to your organs.

And that's when bad things can happen.

No. 2: That's why this stealth killer is linked to so many different diseases—because it affects so many different organs. Every system in your body relies on oxygen and blood flow to survive.

For example, medical experts have believed for years that the neuropathy so many diabetics struggle with is caused by nerve damage. But a recent study from Johns Hopkins published in June 2011 in the journal *Brain* reported that small blood vessel damage may actually be at the root of the excruciating pain, numbness, and tingling that can drive many people with diabetes mad.

In fact, more and more doctors are now beginning to recognize what I've been seeing for years—that microcirculation may hold the key to all things related to aging. As was written in the *Townsend Letter for Doctors and Patients*, "The experts all agree that improving microcirculation is essential to enjoying a long and healthy life." In fact, the same article points out, "The most common thread in premature [aging] is impaired microcirculation."

No. 3: These sorts of blood-vessel-related problems don't just start when you've been diagnosed with a disease like full-blown diabetes. Damage to your small blood vessels can begin well before a diagnosis. For example, you're putting your small blood vessels at risk each day your blood sugar starts to elevate, even if you don't have diabetes.

Every time you eat a meal that is filled with a lot of simple carbohydrates—i.e., any white breads, pasta, etc. (you know, the usual American diet)—it destroys your blood vessels, slowly but surely.

So focusing on your food choices should certainly be your first priority. Yes, you'll probably have to make some changes. That's the bad news... the GOOD news is, making those changes doesn't have to be so hard.

And you don't have to go out and buy anything special. In fact, you can start today—at your next meal, even—with things you already have in your kitchen.

For example, one of my favorite ways to fill up without reaching for the bread basket is to begin each meal with a savory vegetable appetizer. Here's one of my go-to, quick, easy recipes:

Blanche some veggies—green beans, broccoli...whatever you've got in the fridge (lightly steam them for 30 seconds or so, then run cold water over them). And then just dip them in rich cream cheese, ranch dressing, peanut butter, or sour cream.

That's what my New Hamptons Health Miracle is all about—simple, easy ways to indulge your way to amazing health...and healthy blood vessels. (Check out Part IV for more great healthy recipes!) And in the meantime, to support those efforts, there are also a handful of nutrients that can help...

Speed healing with this "triple-threat cure"

There are many nutrients that work to support blood flow and blood-vessel health. But I have three favorites that all have research behind them to support their role in supporting small blood-vessel health in particular.

Triple-threat player No. 1

If I had to choose my favorite supplement for blood vessel support (and just about everything else, for that matter), it would have to be *Pycnogenol®*.

Pycnogenol is an extract from the bark of a particular type of pine tree that only grows along the southwest coast of France, in the Les Landes de Gascogne area.

Since researchers began looking at it more closely over 60 years ago, more than 220 studies have been published on the benefits of Pycnogenol—demonstrating its antioxidant properties, its ability to help reduce blood sugar, and its effects on cardiovascular and circulatory health. And clinical research has shown that one of the primary ways Pycnogenol benefits your circulation is by targeting collagen and elastin, which are the building blocks that line your blood vessels.

Unfortunately, a combination of aging and less-than-ideal food choices cause collagen and elastin to break down. But Pycnogenol helps the body replenish these two critical substances—and keeps your blood vessels working the way they're supposed to in the process.

It's something that everyone can benefit from, and I recommend 50 to 100 mg a day for general health. If you have diabetes or blood sugar concerns, you may need additional support. I have my diabetes patients take 100 to 200 mg of Pycnogenol per day.

Fortunately, given the strong research behind this product, Pycnogenol is readily available in most vitamin retail shops like GNC or health-food stores like Whole Foods. It is also easily found online. And while it is on the expensive side relatively speaking, it's because Pycnogenol comes from only one, proprietary source/supplier.

And that's actually a good thing, because you can always count on the quality of the product. The company that makes Pycnogenol is among the best in the business—with top-notch dedication to quality and science. So regardless of the brand you purchase, just be sure it has the name Pycnogenol listed on the ingredient label.

Triple-threat player No. 2

Resveratrol appears to help keep blood vessels healthy by stimulating nitric oxide synthase activity. Which is simply a fancy way of saying it helps to keep the blood vessels open. It may also help keep blood platelets from sticking together, so blood flows more smoothly. The same reason your physician probably recommends that you take an aspirin each day. But there are some significant risks associated with daily aspirin intake. Resveratrol can have a similar affect without the risk.

Of course, I'm sure you've heard you can get the benefits of resveratrol by drinking red wine. However, due to the high sugar content of red wine, you're better off getting resveratrol from a supplement. I recommend 500 mg per day of resveratrol.

And again, thanks to the growing volume of research on the benefits of resveratrol, it is readily available in most vitamin retailers and online. Just make sure to look for trans-resveratrol, which is the most potent and active form.

Triple-threat player No. 3

Diosmin is an antioxidant and anti-inflammatory ingredient found mainly in citrus fruits. Technically speaking, it's a bioflavonoid that is closely related to other citrus bioflavonoids like rutin, quercetin, and hesperidin. In fact, Diosmin and hesperidin are often used in combination to support the circulatory system and treat heart disease and are used widely in Europe for varicose veins and hemorrhoids. One study showed that Diosmin helps repair microcirculation and blood vessel function throughout the body. This resulted in less edema—a sign that kidney function was improving.

Diosmin is most commonly taken on a short-term basis to relieve varicose veins and hemorrhoids. So you will likely find it in combination products geared toward those conditions.

Such products tend to have higher dosages (450-900 mg to be taken up to twice a day for a few days). However, it can be beneficial if taken in lower levels to help promote healthy blood vessel health ongoing.

Other blood-vessel-supporting supplements that I recommend to my patients include **pomegranate** and an herb called **butcher's broom**.

Surprising symptoms of small blood vessel disease

Take a look at the following list. If any of these symptoms sound familiar, your small blood vessels may be the culprit...

- Cold hands and feet
- Feeling cold all the time
- Numbness or tingling in the hands or feet
- Blurred vision
- Skin bruising that doesn't heal quickly
- Frequent urination
- Persistent dark under-eye circles (despite getting adequate sleep)
- Leg and/or toe cramping

Pomegranate and butcher's broom have been used for centuries in supporting leg and vein health. Science is finally catching up and starting to understand the mechanisms behind why these nutrients work—and the research is very exciting.

Between easy mealtime swaps to keep your blood sugar balanced (and, in turn, keep it from wreaking havoc on your circulation), and the added support of the triple-threat cure of Pycnogenol, resveratrol, and Diosmin, you'll keep your blood vessels healthy without having to give it a second thought.

Simple as that.

Warning: The essential nutrient 50% of Baby Boomers aren't getting enough of

According to current estimates, 1 out of every 2 Americans over the age of 60 have metabolic syndrome. And unfortunately that number seems to be growing every day. Which is why this next tip is especially important.

Researchers found that people with metabolic syndrome are much more likely to be deficient in vitamin E than people who don't suffer from this all-too-common condition.

Metabolic syndrome is a condition characterized by high concentrations of fat in the abdomen, obesity, elevated triglycerides, high blood pressure, high fasting blood glucose, and low HDL cholesterol. And it's often a gateway to serious health issues.

The study involved 20 people—10 with metabolic syndrome and 10 without. Each group was given 15 mg of vitamin E.

Blood tests 72 hours later showed that the group without metabolic syndrome absorbed an average of almost 30% of the vitamin, while the metabolic syndrome group absorbed only 26%.

And the metabolic syndrome group had a maximum vitamin E blood concentration of 2.0 micromoles per liter, compared to 2.7 for the people without metabolic syndrome.

In other words, if you have metabolic syndrome, you won't get as much of this essential nutrient from food or supplements as someone without it—which sets you up for deficiency.

Another reason you need more fat

So why does metabolic syndrome wreak havoc with vitamin E levels?

The researchers think it may be because people with metabolic syndrome have lower levels of two types of lipoproteins that help the body absorb and use E. (And they think the oxidative stress associated with metabolic syndrome could be the reason for the reduced levels of lipoproteins.)

Whether or not you have metabolic syndrome, it's important to make sure you absorb as much of the vitamin E you get from foods and supplements as possible. Since vitamin E is a fat-soluble nutrient, one way to do this is to take your supplements with foods that contain fat.

I recommend taking it with macadamia nut oil. This ultra-nutritious oil is one of the best sources of healthy monounsaturated fat.

And remember, when it comes to vitamin E, all supplements are not created equal. An easy way to make sure you get enough vitamin E every day is to look for a multivitamin that includes 100 IU.

Chapter 15

Cholesterol's "Silent Partner"

A statin-free blueprint for avoiding heart attack and stroke

If there's one thing history has taught us, it's that the wheels of medicine grind at a painfully slow pace.

Up until the mid-nineteenth century it was commonplace for doctors to move from patient to patient, surgery to surgery without once washing their hands.

When a young Hungarian doctor named Ignaz Philipp Semmelweis presented evidence that infection and disease could be greatly reduced by doctor's simply washing their hands between patients, the medical community scoffed. Many even took offense at the suggestion and eventually Semmelweis was laughed out of medicine. It was years after Semmelweis' death in a Hungarian insane asylum that his theory was finally proven correct and slowly implemented into common medical practice.

Likewise, in the 1960's a brilliant doctor and researcher named Albert Sabin invented an oral vaccine for Polio which was superior to the injectable Salk vaccine in three separate ways. Again, the medical community turned a blind eye and Sabin eventually left America to treat patients in Russia, Mexico and Singapore to prove his vaccine's superiority. It took five long years and hundreds of millions of successful inoculations overseas before Sabin's now ubiquitous sugar cube Polio vaccine was finally accepted into widespread medical practice in America.

And now, in the 21st century it appears we're at another medical crossroads in terms of the importance of cholesterol as a major risk factor for heart disease.

Much like the stubborn philosophies that were ingrained in medical thinking of the past, the idea of cholesterol as the foremost predictor of heart attack and stroke is likewise believed and repeated among doctors of today without so much as a second thought.

Further compounding this belief is a modern pharmaceutical industry with a $20 billion yearly stake in the widespread acceptance of cholesterol management as the be-all end-all in terms of avoiding heart attacks and stroke.

But even in the face of such insurmountable odds, studies are coming to light which both directly challenge the overall importance of cholesterol and point to a second and much more dangerous component to heart disease.

Colossal cracks in the case for cholesterol

In 2009, the American Heart Association published a Harvard University study which began to raise eyebrows among enlightened doctors across the country.

The study, one of the largest of its kind, involved 1,315 physicians and over 17,500 men and women in 26 different countries. Though many important findings were made in the study's five years of research, one of the most astonishing facts was something the statin industry would prefer you never heard at all.

Shockingly, the study found that, "of the nearly 1.7 million heart attacks and strokes that occur annually in the United States, more than half occur among apparently healthy men and women with average or low levels of cholesterol."

So there must be another, more important factor involved in heart attacks and stroke that raises risk regardless of cholesterol levels. More on that in a moment.

Another study which raised serious questions as to the importance of cholesterol was the Lyon Diet Heart Study.

The study, also published by the American Heart Association, involved over 400 men and women who had already experienced a heart attack. The participants were split into two groups: A control group which adopted a traditional "heart healthy" diet focused on lowering cholesterol. And an experimental group which adopted an altogether different diet.

To the surprise of mainstream doctors everywhere, after 46 months the group not following the traditional diet managed to lower their overall risk of heart disease between 50%-70% without lowering their cholesterol levels one bit! (I'll discuss the unbelievable way they did this in minute.) These results were so surprising that the doctors involved decided to stop the study early for moral reasons because the risk of heart disease remained so high for the control group.

These two high-profile studies published by the American Heart Association (of all places!) teach us two important things that completely fly in the face of mainstream medical thinking.

1. Even with perfect cholesterol levels the odds of suffering a devastating heart attack or stroke are still over 50%.

2. It is entirely possible to drastically reduce your risk of heart attack and stroke without lowering your cholesterol.

So for now, let's focus on the surprisingly overlooked reason that makes that first statement true and then get into exactly how you can quickly and easily accomplish the second.

Cholesterol's "Silent Partner"

Around the same time that Harvard University published its study revealing that increased cholesterol levels were found in less than 50% of all heart attack and stroke victims, researchers at the World Health Organization published a study which pointed to an overlooked risk factor that seemed to account for the other half.

It was a blood marker known as **fibrinogen**. Now don't feel bad if you've never heard of fibrinogen, most doctors you'll talk to these days likely haven't either. In fact, in their own words, the World Health Organization describes this crucial blood marker as being *"almost forgotten by the clinical community."*

But by publishing this groundbreaking study they hoped to both remind mainstream medicine of the vital importance of this risk factor and set standards for measuring its levels in patients.

Now, to understand just how dangerous excess levels of this blood marker can be we must first look at how it works in your bloodstream.

Anatomy of a heart attack

Fibrinogen is a protein produced by the liver and in small quantities it is an absolutely vital and necessary component for survival.

When you cut or scrape your skin, fibrinogen is the agent which causes the blood to congeal and eventually create a scab which clots the wound altogether. It also works on a molecular level in much the same way, by clotting small stress-related cracks and crevices in your arteries.

The problem begins when levels of fibrinogen become elevated. When this occurs, instead of creating a small clot to repair an artery imperfection, the fibrinogen begins to work overtime creating a much larger clot than is needed. These oversized clots can grow to the point where they close off veins, blood vessels or major arteries entirely and cause devastating heart attacks and stroke.

To put this in simpler terms: A heart attack or stroke is caused by a clot which shuts off blood flow in a vein or artery and a clot is caused by excess fibrinogen. Now to be fair, excess amounts of cholesterol can latch onto these clots making them bigger and speeding the process… but the clot forms regardless of cholesterol levels in the blood.

That is exactly why the World Health Organization study stated that "the risk of high cholesterol levels strongly depends on concomitant high fibrinogen levels. In contrast, the risk calculated for high fibrinogen is fairly independent of the cholesterol concentration."

This is also why the same study concluded that testing for and management of fibrinogen in the bloodstream could be even "more important than cholesterol and lipoproteins."

And this is far from the first study to point out the danger of excess fibrinogen. Another Harvard University Study published in the *Journal of the American College of Cardiology* found that "Those with high fibrinogen levels had a **twofold** increase in myocardial infarction (heart attack) risk."

And still another study published in the prestigious *Royal College of General Practitioners* found that when coupled with other heart-health risk factors such as cholesterol and high blood pressure, "**incidence of heart attacks was respectively six times and 12 times greater** in those with high plasma fibrinogen levels than in those with low fibrinogen levels."

In other words, even if you have high cholesterol or high blood pressure you're respectively 600% and 1200% less likely to suffer a heart attack if your fibrinogen levels are in line!

Which brings us to the main question:

How can you control fibrinogen levels?

Alarmingly, this is a question that mainstream medicine has so far been unable to answer. In fact, the peer reviewed website www.labtestsonline. org states that tests for fibrinogen levels have "not gained widespread acceptance because there are no direct treatments for elevated levels."

Other studies have also found that mainstream clot-busters like aspirin and warfarin have absolutely no effect on fibrinogen levels.

If fact, in my own practice I've found that these drugs actually tend to *increase* fibrinogen levels in patients.

Luckily, however, nature has provided us with a method to quickly and easily control levels of fibrinogen and in turn slash your risk of heart attack and stroke. I'll get to that in a moment, but first let's talk about how to find out if you need this natural intervention at all.

Assessing your risk: The first step to slashing it!

Your levels of fibrinogen can be easily tested by any doctor simply by asking for what's called a *fibrinogen activity test*. Currently, many doctors will only perform this test if you're displaying excessive bleeding (a rare sign of low fibrinogen levels) or if you have already formed a blood clot (the after-effect of excess fibrinogen). However, your doctor should be able to easily add a fibrinogen activity test to your regular blood work. All you have to do is ask!

Generally, I like to see my patients' fibrinogen levels under 300 mg/dl. If your levels are lower, I'd continue to get your levels tested around twice a year. If higher, you should get your levels tested every three months.

But more importantly, if you have high levels of fibrinogen you should take steps to get that number down to acceptable levels.

The cardiovascular cure-all that's stunning science

Years ago, researchers conducted a clinical trial called the Lyon Diet Heart Study. The experimental group in that study was able to lower their overall risk of heart disease by an astonishing 50%-70% without lowering their cholesterol levels. And these were patients who had *already* suffered a heart attack so their risk levels at the beginning of this study were through the roof!

So how did they do it? The experimental group was told to follow a strict Mediterranean diet. And doctors found that the primary reason for the improved health of these participants can be attributed directly to the high levels of Omega-3 fatty acids found in this diet.

So it's no surprise that Omega 3's are one of the only proven natural substances I know of that can quickly and effectively lower your levels of fibrinogen in the bloodstream.

In fact, yet another study published by the American Heart Association found that Omega 3's can lower your levels of this deadly blood marker as much as 13.2%.

And as we discussed earlier, getting your levels of fibrinogen down can lower your overall risk of heart diseases an eye-popping 600%-1200%!

Of course, the heart healthy benefits of Omega 3's don't stop with fibrinogen. The benefits of this fabulous fatty acid are vast and well documented. One meta-analysis which reviewed close to two dozen separate studies on Omega 3's found that this amazing fatty acid improved CRP, Triglycerides, blood pressure and cholesterol levels. But it didn't stop there, Omega 3's were also linked to improvements in depression, memory and even Alzheimer's Disease!

So how do you get more Omega 3s?

First, you can start eating foods which are rich in Omega 3's such as salmon, mackerel and sardines. Also eat plenty of nuts and seeds such as macadamia nuts, pecans, walnuts, and flaxseeds. And use macadamia nut oil, estate-bottled olive oil, and avocado oil.

Also, I always recommend that my patients supplement with 3,000 mg of fish oil daily (one that contains EPA and DHA).

And finally, as per the Lyon Diet Heart Study you can make a significant dent in your fibrinogen levels by following a Mediterranean Diet— which is exactly what my New Hamptons Health Miracle is…only with the added benefit of an emphasis on the use of macadamia nut oil over olive oil. It's the easiest and most enjoyable diet there is to follow, hands down. For all the details, see Part III of this book. This section will provide all the steps to success with my New Hamptons Health Miracle—no matter what your health concerns may be.

Chapter 16

The 72-hour secret to a heart that's
STRONG AS STEEL!

True heart health isn't as complicated as you've been led to believe. In fact, it all boils down to an astonishingly simple secret…

In just a moment, you'll discover the secret to defeating the ONE thing that's secretly contributing to most of your heart problems. You'll get the tips, hints, and details—as well as the encouragement—you need to turn the tables on this overlooked heart killer starting in just 72 hours.

Plus, you'll also discover:

- The heart-health markers way more important than cholesterol

- Six red-flag symptoms you'd never expect—but should never ignore

- Seven easy-to-find natural supplements that can set your heart on a path to healing

- The simple $15.00 test that predicts future heart attacks with 99% accuracy!

- The European pocket-sized device that can boost your odds of surviving a heart attack by 91%

- The free, one-minute heart test you can do right at home

How healthy is your heart?

I discuss the importance of microcirculation—the small blood vessels and capillaries throughout your body—in Chapter 12, The Triple-Threat Cure. Keeping your microcirculatory system healthy is one of the most important things you can do for your overall health. Those small vessels are the lifeline to every point in your body, from head to toe.

But once you've addressed your microcirculation, it's important to turn your attention to the "Big Picture"—your heart and arteries.

Here's what you need to know...

1. This is not a battle between HDL "good" cholesterol vs. LDL "bad" cholesterol. It's not even about total cholesterol. There are far more important markers of heart health than cholesterol.

2. Chest pain isn't the only symptom that can signal a problem.

3. Seven natural supplements can improve heart and artery health—without risky side effects.

4. It all boils down to one simple secret to promoting a heart that's strong as steel in just 72 hours.

But first, there's one aspect involved in heart health that is still overshadowed by the mainstream's incessant focus on cholesterol...

The heart risk the "experts" aren't warning you about

Inflammation plays a huge role in this risk picture. The inflammatory process can take a toll on your heart and blood vessels. Chronic inflammation damages artery walls. That damage gives them a rougher surface. And that gives a foothold for plaque to latch on to.

Then the plaque continues to build up, which narrows arteries. And prevents blood from flowing freely. In turn, your blood pressure goes up. And your risk of potentially fatal stroke-inducing blood clots goes up, too.

But the big question is...

How can you tell if this is happening to your heart and arteries? How can you tell if they're healthy or not?

Six surprising symptoms of heart problems

Sure, chest pain is a big red flag of a heart attack. But it's also one of the last signs. And sometimes it never occurs at all.

The truth is, there are many more symptoms that can indicate the heart isn't as healthy as it could be. And these can occur well before an actual heart attack. Which gives you more time to correct the underlying problems...and avoid a heart attack altogether.

A few of the most surprising symptoms include:

- *Neck, jaw, throat, or ear pain.* Damaged heart tissue can send pain signals up and down the spinal cord to nerves that radiate out to these areas.

- *Swollen feet or ankles.* When you take off your socks, do you see an indent or mark where the elastic band at the top touched your ankle or calf? If so, it may indicate that your heart isn't pumping effectively, allowing fluid to leak out from your blood vessels.

- *Hair loss.* Men who are losing or have lost hair at the crown of the head have a 23% higher risk of heart disease.

- *Yellow bumps on the skin.* Technically, these are called "xanthomas" and they can be a sign of high triglycerides.

- *Frequent urination.* Most people assume this is a symptom of diabetes. And it can be. But it can also result from decreased blood flow from the heart to the kidneys.

- *Coughing at night.* This can signal a buildup of fluid in the chest and heart that occurs when you lie flat at night.

Of course, these symptoms may have other causes, too. But if you have more than one, or if it doesn't go away within a few days, it's a good idea to get a full heart workup done.

There are a handful of time-tested medical tests that can track heart rate, blood flow, and heart function. And, scientists have honed in on several blood tests that can help you monitor your heart and artery health. There's also solid research that support some easy-to-find nutritional supplements to protect, strengthen, and improve the markers that threaten your circulatory system. So let's start with...

Three tests I use to monitor my own heart health

EKG (Electrocardiogram). An EKG is a simple, painless test. It usually takes only 5-10 minutes. During an EKG, you'll have electrodes attached to your arms, legs, and chest. The electrodes are attached to a machine that detects and records the heart's electrical activity. It shows how fast the heart is beating and its rhythm, so it can detect signs of heart damage. I recommend getting an EKG every year.

Echocardiogram. An echocardiogram uses sound waves to monitor blood flow. It provides information about the heart's size and shape, and how well the heart and valves are working. During an echocardiogram, you'll lie on a table and an ultrasound technician will press a small, microphone-like "wand" against your chest and move it around slowly. The "wand" (technically called a transducer) sends sound waves into the chest and picks up the echoes as they bounce off various parts of the heart. The echoes are sent to a video monitor that records pictures of your heart for your doctor to review. I recommend getting an echocardiogram yearly.

Ultrafast computed tomography (CT). An ultrafast CT can take multiple images of the heart in the time it takes for a single heartbeat. It can also detect very small amounts of calcium within the heart and the coronary arteries. So it provides much more detail about heart function, and can detect even very early signs of heart disease. During an ultrafast CT scan, you'll lie on a table that slides into the scanning machine. You'll be asked to lie very still as the scanner rotates around you, generating X-rays that your doctor will review later. You'll hear loud clicking sounds, which are normal. I recommend getting an ultrafast CT scan every five years.

Simple blood tests that show hidden dangers

In addition to the regular scans above, there are six blood markers that can help predict your risk for heart attacks, stroke, and overall cardiovascular disease.

But one important note: Some of these aren't tests that mainstream physicians commonly order. So you may want to bring this list with you to your next appointment, to be sure you're getting a complete picture of your heart.

B-type natriuretic peptide (BNP). BNP is a biomarker of tension in the heart wall. It can be an indicator of heart failure. The higher your level, the worse your risk. You want yours to be below 100.

C-reactive Protein (CRP). The body produces CRP during the inflammation process. In the Harvard Women's Health Study, women with the highest CRP levels were more than four times as likely to die from coronary disease, or to suffer a non-fatal heart attack or stroke, compared to those with lower levels.

- Less than 1.0 = Low risk
- 1.0-2.9 = Intermediate risk
- Greater than 3.0 = High risk

I recommend getting your CRP tested twice per year.

Homocysteine. Research shows that homocysteine can injure the endothelium, or lining of arteries. Homocysteine also contributes to production of pro-inflammatory chemicals called cytokines. And, it promotes oxidation of the fat and LDL cholesterol that can build up in arteries damaged by inflammation.

Elevated levels have been linked with atherosclerosis (artery damage), and higher risk of heart attack, stroke, and dangerous blood clots.

One little-known fact about this blood test: It actually measures the level of B-vitamins in your blood (folic acid, vitamins B12, and B6). If you have a vitamin B deficiency you will have a high homocysteine level. And most Americans are B-vitamin deficient, because processed foods and sugar actually steal these essential nutrients from your body.

I like to see my patients' homocysteine levels at 8 or below. And I recommend having it tested every three months if your first test shows elevated levels. (Or twice per year if they're normal.)

Fibrinogen. Fibrinogen is a sticky protein that promotes blood clots and affects blood "thickness." It can help predict numerous heart risks, including stroke risk and heart attack.

In fact, a decade ago, a large-scale study conducted in Europe showed that "fibrinogen is a powerful predictor of stroke, including fatal and non-fatal strokes, first-time strokes, and hemorrhagic and ischemic strokes."

Another study found that high fibrinogen levels predicted recurrent angina, cardiac catheterization, and major events like heart attack and death.

I like to see this number below 300. If yours is higher, be careful which treatment option you choose (I've outlined the best—and safest—options in the box on page 160).

Get your fibrinogen tested every three months if your first test shows elevated levels. (Or twice per year if they're normal.)

Lipid profile. This test measures levels of fats (lipids) in the bloodstream. A lipid profile will show HDL, LDL, total cholesterol, and—most importantly—triglycerides.

There's also a new test that I've been recommending to my patients, called the Vertical Auto Profile (VAP) Cholesterol Test. It gives you a detailed analysis of HDL and LDL.

You see, your HDL cholesterol may not be all good. And even if your LDL is high, a more detailed analysis can show whether those LDL particles are truly "bad" or not.

That said, keep in mind cholesterol isn't the danger it's been made out to be. And it's not the most important of the heart-health markers. But for the sake of giving you a "barometer" for this particular test, here are the ranges I would look for in a patient:

- Total cholesterol around 200 mg/dL
- HDL-cholesterol 60 mg/dL or higher

- LDL-cholesterol less than 110 mg/dL or lower
- Triglycerides 100 mg/dL or below

Get your lipids tested every three months. But keep in mind, this is more about the total lipid profile. These numbers can't stand alone. In fact, the cholesterol numbers can be higher than the ones I listed above and still be acceptable—IF your triglycerides are low. And if the ratio between HDL to triglycerides is greater than 1.0 and the ratio of total cholesterol to HDL cholesterol is less than 2.5.

Lipoprotein(a). Lipoprotein(a) (or Lp(a), for short) is a substance that builds on the inner lining of arteries, promoting inflammation and damaging artery walls. Lp(a) also contains a blood clotting component, which compounds the risk for heart disease and stroke even further.

You should get your Lp(a) tested every year. And you want your level to be below 10.

Ferritin. This is a seldom-run heart-health test, but it's a critical one. It indicates how much iron is stored in your body. Which is important because excess iron can cause organ damage—and too little can cause heart disease. I recommend having your ferritin level tested yearly if your level is normal. Generally this level should be around 75. If yours is higher or lower than that, you should have follow-up testing done quarterly.

The simple $15.00 test that predicts future heart attacks with 99% accuracy!

What if you could literally see your heart's future? Well, now—with a cheap, two-minute test—you can.

I know, it sounds like science fiction but it's been clinically proven.

Just last year, researchers from the Karolinska Institute in Sweden discovered the secret to determining whether or not you're in imminent danger of having a heart attack.

Most people assume chest pain is a telltale sign of heart attack. And it can be. So this frightening symptom sends thousands of people to the emergency room each year. But chest pain can also result from any number of benign causes, including anxiety and bronchitis. The problem is, ER doctors don't have any reliable methods to rule out heart attack. So these patients are often admitted for further observation. But, many times, it turns out they're totally fine. Which means a significant number of chest-pain related hospital admissions are **completely unnecessary**.

But now you may be able to save yourself the time, expense, and worry.

The Swedish researchers found that patients with chest pain who have no detectable levels of a chemical called "high-sensitivity cardiac troponin T" were at very low risk for a heart attack within the next month.

And the results held even when the researchers adjusted for other risk factors of heart disease. In fact, they found a 99.8 percent probability that people with no detectable levels of this particular blood chemical were not at risk for heart attack.

That's right, 99%!

And this was no small study. They followed over 14,000 people for 2 years to come up with these numbers.

The researchers themselves were blown away by the results. The lead author of the study said "Despite our observations before the study, we were still surprised by the strength of our findings."

But only a *staggeringly* low number of Americans know this test is available to them.

Current clinical guidelines actually recommend that patients should receive this test within three hours after chest pain begins. Unfortunately, many times, doctors wait until after the patient has been admitted to run it.

But the authors of this study estimate that using this simple blood test along with an electrocardiogram screening (ECG) could potentially save between 500 and 1,000 unnecessary admissions in each and every hospital *per year*. Not to mention the fact that it also has the potential to **save hundreds of thousands of lives!**

Of course, even despite the very strong results, doctors caution that more research is needed. And it should be noted, as well, that even if this test indicates you're not at high risk, there is always a small possibility that you could suffer a cardiac event in the following weeks.

However, even with these two caveats, the Swedish researchers' new findings unequivocally support the role of this test in determining cardiac risk.

If you or someone you love experiences chest pain, you should seek emergency care right away. But before you agree to be admitted, ask the attending physician to run the "hs-cTnT assay" (the technical lab term for the "high-sensitivity cardiac troponin T" test) along with an ECG. If your results don't indicate the presence of hs-cTnT or impaired blood flow, it's very likely that you're in the clear.

The European pocket-sized device that can boost your odds of surviving a heart attack by 91%

A staggering 90% of sudden heart attack victims in the U.S. die before they ever reach the hospital.

But there's a cutting-edge device available right now that could flip this sobering statistic *upside down.*

Imagine a portable device you could purchase today that can skyrocket your odds of surviving a sudden cardiac event outside a hospital from **just 5% to over 90%.**

And I'm not talking about a pacemaker that needs to be implanted in your chest or a bulky defibrillator that takes two people to lift off the wall.

This is a battery-powered, portable piece of technology that only requires you to press 3 buttons to save a life.

It's called an Automated External Defibrillator (AED) and it takes the heart-starting power of those "crash carts" you see in hospitals—and condenses it into a convenient, compact unit. Honestly, it's small enough that you could take it with you *anywhere.* It can fit in your glove compartment, your purse or your coat pocket!

In fact, it's so durable and portable that the president even keeps one on hand at the White House and on Air Force One.

And it's so simple even kids can use it easily. According to a study published in the journal *Circulation*, a group of 6th graders using an AED for the first time performed almost on par with trained emergency medical technicians in terms of speed. And they were just as accurate.

Unfortunately, while portable AEDs are common in Europe, most Americans don't even know this simple, life-saving technology exists! Let alone that you can purchase one to protect yourself and your loved ones RIGHT NOW.

There are actually a number of AEDs available. But the smallest, lightest model is called the HeartSine Samaritan® PAD 350P. In the event of a sudden heart attack, a user simply turns on the unit and follows the instructions to help the victim. Audio and visual prompts help the user through each step of the process, from attaching electrode pads to delivering shock (if necessary), and even administering CPR.

As you might guess, this sort of technology doesn't come cheap. Portable AED units can range in price from $1200 to $3000 depending on the source and model you choose. (The HeartSine Samaritan® PAD 350P costs $1,175 and you can find it at www.HeartsineSamaritan.com.) But the protection and peace of mind you get from this investment is truly priceless.

The free, one-minute heart test you can do right at home

I've written before about how your waistline is a clear indicator of your health status. But it's not the only measurement that can tell you whether you're at increased risk of some serious health concerns.

Several studies have shown that there's a significant connection between neck circumference and heart disease.

In fact, researchers have determined that neck circumference is an accurate predictor of risk independent of other factors, like BMI and waist size. In other words, even if you're not carrying around an obvious spare tire around your midsection, you could still be at risk—and measuring your neck may be all it takes to clue you in.

In a recent study, published in November in the *American Journal of Clinical Nutrition*, looked at just over 300 subjects. And researchers found neck circumference was positively associated with blood pressure and triglycerides—especially in women.

Another, even bigger study took place in 2013 in China. Researchers examined 4,200 subjects and had similar findings, with the notable addition of lower HDL (good) cholesterol levels in people with wider necks.

Both of these studies also correlated neck circumference with increased risk of insulin resistance—one of the biggest warning signs impending diabetes. In all instances, the wider a person's neck, the worse their heart health markers were. The same held true with blood sugar control. So get out your trusty tape measure and take a minute to measure your neck.

For men, measurements greater than 14.5 inches are cause for concern. And for women, anything over 13 inches raises a red flag.

If your measurements put you in the "high risk" category, it's definitely worth following up with your doctor to get a complete picture of your heart health.

In the meantime, you can get a head start with my special report, *The World's Easiest Heart Disease Cure*. In it, I detail exactly which tests you need—and which ones you don't—along with safe, natural strategies for protecting and healing your heart.

Kick the No. 1 cause of heart disease— starting in just 72 hours!

When it comes to keeping your heart humming on all cylinders, here's what you need to know…the cause of heart disease essentially boils down to ONE thing.

That's right—just ONE simple secret: SUGAR.

If you haven't already given up sugar, now is the time.

Seven heart supplements everyone should be taking

These seven supplements will help support every important aspect of heart health. They're all easy to find, so there's simply no reason not to take them on a daily basis.

CoEnzyme Q10 (CoQ10). I recommend a CoQ10 supplement—100 to 600 mg daily. The dosage will vary depending on whether you already have heart disease (higher dose) or are preventing it (lower dose).

Omega-3 Fish oil. I recommend 3,000 mg of fish oil daily (one that contains both EPA and DHA fatty acids).

Folate & B-vitamins. Take at least a B100 complex. However, to really improve your homocysteine levels, you need at least 2,000 mcg of B12, 5 mg of folic acid, and 100 mg of B6 per day. Oh, and if you enjoy an occasional cocktail—which is perfectly fine—just keep in mind that alcohol does deplete B vitamins, so you will need more of all the "Bs."

Nattokinase. Nattokinase is an extract derived from Japanese fermented soybeans. I recommend 1,000 to 3,000 fibrin units per day (3,000 fibrin units equals roughly 150 mg).

Pycnogenol. I recommend a 100 mg daily dose of Pycnogenol for optimal heart health.

Resveratrol. I recommend 500 mg of resveratrol daily.

Vitamin D. I recommend at least 2,000-5,000 IU per day of vitamin D3 (the active form of the nutrient). And be sure to get your blood levels of 25 hydroxy vitamin D checked periodically by your physician. This is the most critical of the vitamin D levels. And I like to see my patients' between 80 and 100.

Sugar is the No. 1 cause of oxidative stress on your heart and arteries. The No. 1 trigger for damaging inflammation. The No. 1 cause of heart disease.

And don't forget that regular table sugar is only one source. High fructose corn syrup is another (look for it on package labels). Simple carbohydrates—potatoes, rice, pastries, jams, crackers, cereals, candy bars, cookies—are also sources. They all need to go.

Think you can't live without sugar? Well I think you can. In fact, I know you can. And I've helped thousands of others do it…starting with this one simple technique.

All it takes is 72 hours. That's it. Imagine, 72 hours from now, you'll be well on your way to living heart-disease-free and even diabetes-free for the rest of your life.

So isn't it worth a shot?

I've seen even the most diehard sugar addicts succeed. Just remember to take it day by day. Don't try to make all your changes at once, keep it easy. Make one change at a time, and in just 72 hours you'll be reformed—for good!

Ready to get started?

Day 1: Cut the crud

This first day is simple: Just avoid everything that you know has sugar without even having to think about it. Cookies, cakes, ice cream, soda— toss them all. If it seems like just one small sweet won't hurt you, try looking at the sweet and visualizing all the sugar it contains. An ounce of hard candy? Picture a 5-teaspoon mound of sugar! A slice of cherry pie? Make that 10 teaspoons. Now imagine sitting down and eating that mound of sugar, and you'll see just how damaging those sweets really are!

Day 2: Un-refine your diet

Get rid of all the processed, refined, and simple carbohydrates in your diet. This means white rice, white flour, sugar, corn syrup, and fruit juice (did you know apple juice has more grams of sugar than a soda?). Whole grains (quinoa, brown rice, and millet, for example) are A-OK.

Day 3: A sugar by any other name

So you switched to whole wheat bread. Great! But did you read the label to make sure it didn't have any simple sugars? You should—and don't just trust the marketing claims, such as "no sugar added." It's surprising how many seemingly safe foods hide sugar, corn syrup, and refined carbohydrates. Take a close look at the ingredients list and avoid sugar, obviously, but also these ingredients:

- Honey
- Concentrated fruit juice
- Barley malt
- Maple syrup
- Rice syrup
- Cane sugar
- Fructose
- Anything that ends in -ose or -ol

Now here's the part where I get the most raised eyebrows, but hear me out:

I need you to give up fruit on day three. Fruit is largely sugar (did you know a banana has 6 grams of sugar?) and therefore needs to be included in the sugar-elimination challenge.

This isn't forever—just until your metabolic imbalances have been corrected, at which point you can add low-sugar fruits like melons and berries back in.

Now don't stop!

Once you're through the first three days, you've made it past the hardest part. So even if you don't feel great just yet, you will—as long as you continue to stick with it. Your body has begun to re-adjust its metabolism. Instead of using sugar for energy, it uses the other food that you feed it for energy—and best of all it is beginning to burn your fat cells as well.

Before you get too depressed over what you can't eat...revel in what you CAN.

You don't need to be afraid of saturated fat. Its role in heart disease is way over-stated. Which means you can enjoy that thick, deliciously marbled steak, or that juicy cheeseburger without worrying. And go ahead and enjoy some cheese on those veggies! There are so many delicious hard cheeses to choose from...and let's face it, cheese just makes everything more fun.

Just make sure you also get plenty of the following:

- Omega-3 fatty fish like salmon, tuna, and mackerel.

- Monounsaturated fatty acids (MUFAs), from sources like macadamia nut oil, estate-bottled olive oil, nuts (almonds, walnuts, macadamias), and avocados.Fresh, non-starchy vegetables—spinach, broccoli, bell peppers, kale, collard greens, string beans, cabbage.

- Whole grains like quinoa, millet, spelt, teff, etc.

And don't stress out over calories. When you're eating the right foods— you'll naturally feel full sooner, and simply stop when you should. No need to drive yourself crazy with all that calorie counting!

Last, but certainly not least...

You knew I would say it. You've got to get moving. No getting around it.

It's a sure-fire way to decrease damaging inflammation. And the best therapy to cut your risk of heart disease, heart attack, and stroke.

Not to mention that exercise will help you lose weight, which helps ease inflammation even further. You don't have to kill yourself, even a little bit will help. Get out after dinner, and get a 15-minute brisk walk. Make it a daily habit...and you'll add years to your life.

Crush Your Cravings

It's 3 o'clock and you've got only one thing on your mind: a chocolate bar. You're pretty sure you're not going to make it through the day without one. Or three. What do you do to get your mind back on track?

Take some glutamine! This protein building-block is a surefire cure for sugar cravings. Take 500 mg (up to three times per day), and you'll watch your sugar cravings disappear.

Chocolate bar? What chocolate bar?

Chapter 17

Natural secrets to reverse Alzheimer's disease and strengthen your brain

After decades of research and billions of dollars spent, mainstream medicine has come up empty-handed on Alzheimer's.

The best you can hope for is delaying symptoms for a year or two… if you're lucky.

Why? Because they've missed the forest for the trees…

They're so hung up on plaques and tangles that they've utterly ignored the most obvious symptom of Alzheimer's that shows up 10 years *before* the disease really starts to take hold.

I'm talking about brain shrinkage.

It's a fact, a brain riddled with Alzheimer's shrinks up like a grape in the summer sun…utterly devastating areas involved in thinking, planning and memory.

And mainstream medicine has no drugs, treatments, or therapies to combat it.

Just recently, an Oxford University study proved that a "pennies-per-day" all-natural cocktail of three simple B vitamins can halt brain shrinkage in its tracks.

The astonishing results, published in the renowned medical journal *The Proceedings of the National Academy of Sciences*, showed that patients with mild to moderate brain shrinkage who took vitamin B6, vitamin B12, and folic acid <u>slowed brain shrinkage by an unheard of 90%!</u>

Yes, I said **90%!** Put simply, this treatment is pulling patients back from the abyss of Alzheimer's.

And if that sounds crazy to you, I can assure you no one was more surprised than the researchers themselves…

Even senior author of the study, A. David Smith was caught totally off guard, saying, "It's a big effect, much bigger than we would have dreamt of, I find the specificity of this staggering."

And it's an effect you can see with your own eyes.

Researchers took MRI scans of patients' brains and highlighted the specific areas that were protected by this natural cocktail…and amazingly, they all lined up perfectly with areas normally ravaged by Alzheimer's disease.

After viewing the MRIs, Paul Thompson, professor of neurology and head of the Imaging Genetics Center at UCLA School of Medicine said, "I've never seen results from brain scans showing this level of protection."

In fact, the only thing more impressive is the effect these three, simple B vitamins have on memory.

An earlier study performed in 2012 showed that patients taking vitamin B6, B12, and folic acid trounced their placebo-taking peers by a whopping 69% on memory tests!

As lead researcher David Smith of Oxford University put it…

"It's the first and only disease-modifying treatment that's worked."

And with rates of Alzheimer's expected to skyrocket in the coming years to 115 million Americans (or 1 in 3)…it couldn't have come along at a better time!

Jess Smith, a communications officer for the U.K. Alzheimer's Society, says this simple treatment has the power to "halve the number of people dying from [Alzheimer's]."

But don't expect your doctor to recommend *anything* but pharmaceuticals anytime soon…Why? Because the money generated from Band-Aid-like Alzheimer's drugs adds up to over $600 billion dollars a year. Put another way, **Alzheimer's disease is simply _too big to cure_**. And as you've seen—it's only going to get bigger.

Pharmaceutical companies (and the FDA who gets paid to approve their products) simply have too much to lose by publicizing a pennies-per-day natural treatment with the potential to wipe out Alzheimer's for good.

But if you or a loved one are suffering from Alzheimer's, you don't have to wait! I've seen in my own patients the remarkable effects these three simple B vitamins can have on cognitive function—and on overall health. So if you're not already supplementing with B vitamins, it's time to get started.

The doses used in the studies were:

- 0.5 milligrams of vitamin B12
  (equivalent to 500 micrograms)

- 20 milligrams of B6

- 0.8 milligrams of folic acid
  (equivalent to 800 micrograms)

You can get quality B vitamin supplements in any natural food store or vitamin shop, as well as from online supplement retailers. And upping your intake of foods rich in these nutrients certainly won't hurt either.

But there's another way to give your brain even more protection from the ravages of Alzheimer's. This one is equally simple—and completely free!

- Vitamin B2: Fish, poultry, meat, and eggs (clams and liver are particularly rich in this nutrient)

- Vitamin B6: Tuna, chicken, turkey, and cantaloupe

- Folic Acid: Spinach and other dark green leafy vegetables

A little exercise leads to big brain benefits

According to four new studies presented at the 2012 Alzheimer's Association International Conference in Vancouver, exercise may be one of the best ways to protect yourself from Alzheimer's.

One of the studies involved 120 sedentary adults without dementia. Half of them were assigned to a walking group. The other half did stretching exercises. A year later, each volunteer had their brain's hippocampus (the memory region) measured with an MRI.

After just one year, the size of the hippocampus increased by 2 percent in the walking group. This is significant because, as I mentioned above, brain shrinkage is one of the hallmarks of Alzheimer's.

Another study found that resistance training (also called weight training, or strength training) led to improvements in three brain regions involving memory. You can get these effects at home by lifting some 5-pound weights while you watch TV. Twice a week—that's all you need.

This research reaffirms what I've been advising my patients for YEARS now. You can stave off all sorts of serious chronic diseases—including dementia—with just a little bit of effort every day. And you don't have to spend hours in the gym. In fact, you don't even have to break a sweat.

Just a simple walk every day, and some light weight training a couple of times a week. That's all it takes to protect your body—and your mind.

Five Alzheimer's-squashing foods you probably have in your kitchen right now

Alzheimer's disease is overtaking the country. And health experts worldwide have been spinning their wheels trying to figure out why.

But I can't stress this enough... There is absolutely NO REASON to wait for the "cocktail of Alzheimer's drugs" that's supposed to come down the pike some 15 years from now. (According to government estimates.)

Thanks to this new research, reversing the process that triggers Alzheimer's disease has never been more possible. And you can start today. In fact, there are some foods you probably have in your kitchen right now that have impressive research supporting their anti-Alzheimer's benefits. These foods are the simplest way to support your brain—starting today.

#1: Eggs

Eggs may be the perfect anti-Alzheimer's food. They're literally packed with brain-supporting nutrients. Starting with cholesterol. Yes, you read that right. As terrified as everyone is of cholesterol (thanks to mainstream medicine), it's actually an essential nutrient for your brain. In fact, high levels of cholesterol have been linked to better memory and mood in healthy middle-aged and elderly people. And higher levels of total cholesterol are associated with a decreased risk of dementia in elderly people.

Eggs are also rich in vitamin A which feeds the hippocampus, the brain region that breeds new brain cells.

And eggs are terrific sources of choline, a nutrient that supports the brain's message relay system (the synapses). Choline also maintains the structure of brain cell membranes.

In a gold-standard randomized study in *Clinical Therapeutics*, dementia patients who took choline had consistent cognitive improvement. And a major review of 10 studies found that choline significantly improved dementia patients' clinical conditions.

#2: Berries

All berries are packed with antioxidants. And one recent study found low blood levels of several key antioxidants in the brains of 41 Alzheimer's patients. That list includes vitamins A and E, lutein, zeaxanthin, lycopene, alpha- and beta-carotene (which are converted into vitamin A in the body).

But blueberries appear to be especially powerful brain-boosters. A study in the journal Subcellular Biochemistry found that the complex mix of polyphenols found specifically in blueberries has beneficial effects on cell signaling and brain cell communication.

#3: Butter

Butter is an excellent source of vitamin A. And vitamin A supports enzymes that create neurotransmitters like dopamine and their receptors.

These are key players in the basic biochemistry of memory. But keep in mind we're talking about real butter, not margarine. And certainly not those blends that claim to be "better" than butter—hardly!

#4: *Sunflower seeds*

Sunflower seeds provide magnesium, a mineral that protects your brain from ammonia (a waste product) and improves memory and learning. A study in the *Journal of Alzheimer's Disease* also found that magnesium helps to decrease levels of the amyloid-beta proteins that lead to Alzheimer's.

They also contain vitamin E. This essential nutrient has all sorts of functions in the body. But it's especially critical for protecting omega-3 fats, which are concentrated in neurons. And a recent study in the *Journal of Alzheimer's Disease* found that dietary intake of vitamin E particularly lowered the risk of dementia.

#5: *Salmon*

Salmon is one of the best sources of omega- 3s that feed and protect your brain's neurons. And one scientific review published in the *Proceedings of the Nutrition Society* found that omega-3 fats from fish significantly protect the brain from dementia.

Protect yourself from Alzheimer's while you sleep

As I've said, sleep is a critical component of health. The benefits go well beyond just feeling physically alert on a daily basis. Unfortunately, it's often overlooked in our always-on-the-go world.

But that quality of sleep is just as important as quantity. And getting uninterrupted rest is just as critical as clocking in the right number of hours. In fact, a recent study indicates that people have trouble sleeping through the night have a higher Alzheimer's risk than those who don't.

The researchers studied older men, who were initially 50 years old, between the years 1970 and 2010. (Yes, a 40-year follow-up period— talk about thorough.) Self-reported sleep disturbances were shown

Heart test predicts dementia

It's hard to imagine a heart disease test could predict your risk of dementia better than an actual dementia test. But according to recent research, this is one fact you can file under "strange-but-true."

Researchers looked at British subjects from the Whitehall II cohort study, all with an average age of around 55 years old.[39] They compared Framingham heart disease and stroke risk scores—a popular test to gauge 10-year heart risk—with Cardiovascular Risk Factors, Aging and Dementia (CAIDE) risk scores. (This latter test estimates dementia risk based on a number of midlife risk factors.)

Subjects took cognitive tests that covered factors like memory, vocabulary, and reasoning skills three different times over the 10-year follow-up.

At decade's end, high heart disease and stroke risk scores translated to cognitive decline in almost every area.

Ultimately, heart test results were stronger predictors of later mental decline.

So what's the bottom line? The secret to a sharp mind lies, quite literally, in your heart.

to increase Alzheimer's risk by 1.5 fold (or 50 percent). And that risk increased with age.

We know that a good night's rest supports brain health in general. But now we can go one step further, to recommend getting your zzz's as a possible guard against Alzheimer's.

Just as interesting: in an earlier article, the same researchers noted that just one night of sleep deprivation (this time in young men) increased levels of molecules that typically show up in cases of brain damage.

I realize, of course, that getting a good night's sleep may be easier said than done for many people. After all, doctors doled out more than 60 million prescriptions for sleep aids in 2011 alone.

But turning to Ambien or one of its over-the-counter cousins isn't the best solution. Because chances are, your insomnia is actually just a symptom of a much bigger underlying issue.

If you have trouble sleeping, you can refer back to Chapter 5: The silent enemy that's stealing your sleep for some insight into what might be causing your restlessness—and what you can do about it.

A huge leap forward in the fight against Alzheimer's

This news is new and it's **huge**. For over a quarter century researchers have been getting Alzheimer's disease wrong. For years they've been focusing all their attention on a sticky, toxic substance that can build up in the brain… beta amyloid plaque.

Billions of dollars have been spent by pharmaceutical companies to find a way to clear or slow the buildup of this plaque in the brain. And it's been seen as the sole "boogey man" responsible for the disease's rapid destruction of memory and the brain.

But a new, large-scale study just published by the Mayo Clinic found that higher amounts of amyloid beta build up in the brain did not correspond to greater levels of mental impairment. In fact, they found that many people can have large amounts of amyloid beta built up in their brain and be *completely free* of Alzheimer's disease.

After decades of research, this 2015 study has finally revealed THE true culprit behind Alzheimer's disease

It's a completely different protein that doesn't simply cause communication problems between neurons like amyloid beta, but actually kills the neurons outright.

A toxic protein known as Tau.

And unlike amyloid beta which is found in healthy patients' brains, Tau is only found in patients with Alzheimer's disease. And, the progression of the disease increases along with the level of Tau in the brain.

For decades pharmaceutical companies have been creating drugs solely focused on clearing amyloid beta from the brain… and they've gotten absolutely nowhere in stopping the disease. That's because they've been overlooking the true cause of this devastating illness this whole time.

Now that it's been found, you can bet pharmaceutical companies will be falling over themselves to create the next Tau-clearing drug. But guess what…

Natural medicine has already found a method of clearing this dangerous Alzheimer's trigger and you can have it in your hands today!

And it all starts with omega-3 fatty acids.

I have been recommending omega-3 fatty acids for decades. Unlike many mainstream drugs designed to treat Alzheimer's that can't seem to get past your body's blood-brain barrier…

Scientific studies have shown that omega-3s are able to target the brain directly and quickly lower your levels of Tau… the true hidden cause of Alzheimer's disease. And this is leading to amazing results…

A 2006 study showed that a diet high in omega-3 fatty acids helped patients lower their Alzheimer's risk by 40 percent.

A more recent 2009 study showed you can **lower your Alzheimer's risk by up to an amazing 67 percent** by simply increasing the amount of omega-3s in your diet!

But things get even more impressive when omega-3s are included in an overall, targeted lifestyle and nutritional protocol for those who are already showing symptoms of Alzheimer's. For many patients it's a night and day difference.

Jan Pierce started experiencing the telltale symptoms of Alzheimer's in her late 60's. She would get lost on once-familiar roads near her house, was unable to remember simple 4-digit numbers, and was unable to remember information she had just read moments before…

She went to see her doctor and was told there was nothing she could do.

But after seeing her mother suffer from the same symptoms, she was determined to find something. She eventually enrolled in a small study using methods similar to those I prescribe, including the natural Tau-clearing breakthrough…

After 3 months she was able to remember phone numbers and navigate and write complex reports without a problem.

Amazingly she was symptom-free!

But she wasn't the only one.

Nine out of 10 patients involved in this small study all experienced similar, incredible results. In fact, 6 of the patients who had to stop working due to their symptoms were able to return to work after three months.

To put these results into perspective…

This was the first time any treatment has had success in reversing Alzheimer's symptoms… ever.

The results were published in the world-renowned medical journal *Aging* just recently.

But I have been recommending these techniques for decades.

Along with a healthy dose of omega-3s, the patients involved in this groundbreaking study were able to reduce their Alzheimer's symptoms by using a variety of natural supplements and lifestyle techniques… many of which you've already heard about in this book.

While each of their therapeutic programs were individualized, following are the key common recommendations they followed:

- Elimination of all simple carbohydrates and processed foods

- Focus on organic lean sources of protein and non-farm-raised fish

- Increased intake of vegetables and fruits

- Reduced stress through yoga, meditation, relaxation techniques

- Increased sleep (close to 8 hours a night)

- Supplementation with fish oil for omega-3 fatty acids (up to 2,000 IUs of EPA/DHA)

- Supplementation with vitamin D3 (2,000 IU)

- Supplementation with B vitamins (including 1 mg of B12 in the form of methylcobalamin)

- Supplementation with coenzyme Q10 (200 mg)

- Supplementation with pre- and probiotics

- Exercise for 30 minutes 4 to 6 days per week

The simple "no-bake dessert" that can knock 2 to 3 decades off your brain's age

Two new studies report that cocoa flavonols can actually reverse cognitive decline and memory loss in older adults.

For the first study, researchers gathered 90 people, ages 65 to 80, who had mild cognitive impairment but not dementia.

Those who drank a chocolate beverage every day scored better on cognition and verbal fluency tests eight weeks later. And they also had lower blood pressure and insulin resistance (a risk factor for diabetes).

The second study, which involved 37 people ages 50 to 69, found that the participants who consumed a chocolate drink every day for three months scored better on memory tests at the end of the study.

"If a participant had the memory of a typical 60-year-old at the beginning of the study, after three months that person on average had the memory of a typical 30- or 40-year-old," said lead study author Dr. Scott Small of the Columbia University Medical Center.

Of course, it's critical to be judicious about the type of chocolate you choose.

Look for dark chocolate that's at least 80 to 90 percent cacao. But if you want the most health benefits, I recommend going for 100 percent cocoa powder.

Is it going to taste good? Not by itself. But that's easy to fix.

Just mix it with unsweetened almond or coconut milk, along with a little bit of stevia (just enough to cut the bitterness). The resulting beverage is one of my favorite "no-bake" desserts. Healthy, simple… and most definitely delicious.

Quick tip to prevent Parkinson's disease

Countless studies point to the health benefits of the flavonoids in berries. Blueberries, strawberries, cranberries. They're all jam-packed with all-important flavonoids called anthocyanins, which give the berries their color.

Now, important research in the journal Neurology shows that berries may help offset the risk of Parkinson's disease.

The Harvard researchers analyzed data from the well-regarded Nurses' Health Study (80,336 women) and the Health Professional Follow-Up Study (49,281 men). They looked at flavonoid-rich food intake in 805 participants who developed Parkinson's disease. And compared it against men and women who did not develop this debilitating disease.

The tally? Men and women who ate the most berries (twice or more every week) had less risk of Parkinson's. Men had the greatest benefit. Those who regularly ate all sorts of foods with flavonoids—tea, berries, apples, and red wine—had 40% less risk of Parkinson's.

So be sure to stock up on plenty of fresh berries at your local farmer's market. They're great with your morning eggs, tossed in a salad, or as a simple dessert with heavy cream.

Slash your risk of Parkinson's by 30% with peppers

New research shows that filling up on nightshades—and peppers in particular—could leave you less vulnerable to Parkinson's disease.

This population study looked at nearly 500 newly diagnosed Parkinson's patients and more than 600 neurologically healthy controls. Researchers found that risk for the disease was inversely associated with consumption of all edible nightshades—including potatoes, tomatoes, and peppers. But not with consumption of any other type of vegetable.

The link was particularly prominent with pepper consumption. In fact, results showed that eating peppers two to four times a week was associated with a 30 percent lower risk of Parkinson's disease.

So what's behind this benefit? Well, it makes even more sense when you consider the anti-Parkinson's power of another member of the nightshade family: tobacco.

This may surprise you, but previous research has shown on a pretty consistent basis that tobacco use—in the form of regular cigarette smoking, and even secondhand smoke—actually lowers Parkinson's risk.

Animal studies suggest that nicotine—an alkaloid in nightshades—may have a neuro-protective effect. This explains why eating nicotine-containing nightshade vegetables appears to carry a similar benefit.

You read that right. Peppers contain nicotine. And this study suggests the more nicotine you get from these vegetables, the stronger your protection. But with an obvious perk: They deliver the goods without the considerable risks of smoking.

In addition to nicotine, peppers are full of vitamin C, flavonoids, and carotenoids—all powerful antioxidants that can help combat inflammation.

Why nightshades aren't as shady as you think

For a lot of people, the word "nightshade" throws up an immediate red flag. It just sounds suspect, doesn't it?

In reality, though, nightshades are simply plants in the Solanaceae family. Along with peppers, this includes vegetables like tomatoes, potatoes, and eggplant—hardly the sinister villains their name evokes.

That isn't to say the bad reputation is completely unwarranted. Because the fact is, nightshade vegetables can be problematic. Specifically, they contain an alkaloid called solanine. Nightshades generate this substance as a natural fungicide and pesticide. And in huge quantities, yes…it can be toxic.

Potatoes with green spots and eyes are a particularly common source of solanine. (That's why it's usually best to discard them. In fact, while you're at it, toss the rest of the sack as well. Starchy potatoes aren't doing you any favors anyway—solanine or not.)

On the whole, though, nightshade foods contain relatively small amounts of this compound. And cooking can cut this already low content in half.

Still, are nightshades inflammatory? For some people, without question. And if you're struggling with arthritis, you could be one of them. But it is absolutely worth your time and effort to determine once and for all if they actually do cause a problem for you. Because if you can eat them, you should.

Try adding them back into your diet. If you notice a flare up of symptoms, cut them back out. If you don't notice a change, then by all means, enjoy as much as you'd like.

The 20-minute habit that can improve Parkinson's symptoms

According to a study in the journal Neurology, people with mild to moderate Parkinson's disease who routinely walk can experience some impressive benefits.

For six months, participants walked three times a week for 45 minutes a pop. According to the researchers, brisk walking:

- Improved motor function and mood by 15 percent
- Increased attention/response control scores by 15 percent
- Increased aerobic fitness and gait speed by 7 percent
- Reduced fatigue by 11 percent

Participants' motor function also improved—by 2.8 points on average.

Here's a short list of common foods in the Solanaceae family

- Sweet and hot peppers
- Eggplant
- Potato
- Tomato
- Tomatillo
- Pepino
- Pimento

- Gooseberry
- Goji berry
- Cayenne
- Chili powder
- Curry powder
- Paprika

(It may not sound like much, but that's actually a clinically significant improvement for Parkinson's patients.)

The study authors concluded that people with mild or moderate Parkinson's who are able to walk unassisted can safely follow the recommended exercise guidelines for healthy adults.

If you need a reminder, those guidelines call for 150 minutes of moderate intensity aerobic exercise per week. If that sounds overwhelming, let me break it down for you…150 minutes a week is really just a little over 20 minutes a day. And those minutes can add years to your life.

Fight MS with six simple supplements

Multiple sclerosis (MS) is one of medicine's great mysteries. No one is really sure what causes the disease. But there is quite a bit of evidence that people who don't get enough vitamin D may be more susceptible. And now, researchers have also discovered that low levels of other important nutrients may also play a role in the development of the disease.

Specifically, I'm talking about natural substances that help fight inflammation—folate (vitamin B9), vitamin E, magnesium, lutein, zeaxanthin, and quercetin. This makes perfect sense when you consider that MS, like so many other chronic diseases, is an inflammatory disorder.

The eye-opening research was presented at the American Academy of Neurology's annual meeting. It included 27 women with MS and 30 women without the disease who kept track of everything they ate, along with the supplements they took, for a year. The researchers discovered deficiencies in the six key nutrients I mentioned above, but made particular note of two of them: folate and magnesium.

The women with MS got an average of 244 mcg of folate a day, compared to 321 mcg for the healthy women. The recommended daily allowance is 400 mcg, which, like most government RDAs, is woefully low. I recommend 5 mg of folic acid a day in supplement form, along with food sources like spinach, avocado, broccoli, and asparagus.

For magnesium, the women with MS had an average intake of 254 mg, while the healthy women hit 321 mg. The RDA is 320 mg, but that's of the less absorbable types of this mineral—magnesium oxide or citrate. Ideally I recommend highly absorbable magnesium orotate (32 mg a day) or taurate (125 mg). They are more expensive and more difficult to find. But definitely worth it if you are fighting MS.

And you can also get more magnesium from foods like spinach, Swiss chard, salmon, halibut, almonds, and cashews.

How much of the other four nutrients do you need for optimal health? I recommend 2,000 IU of vitamin E, 6 mg of lutein, 4 mg of zeaxanthin, and 50 mg of quercetin.

Chapter 18

1 Hour Memory Breakthrough!
Squash "senior moments"
with the Bavarian Brain Booster

Some doctors dismiss "senior moments." They will tell you memory lapses are a natural part of aging and there's nothing you can do about it. Or they suggest you exercise your brain by doing crossword puzzles… or watching Jeopardy…or memorizing your family's phone numbers.

Don't get me wrong—I'm all for mental workouts. But they're more for the long-term health of your brain.

What if I told you it's possible to substantially improve your memory in just one hour? And that you can keep your focus and concentration strong and steady? And even reduce stress and improve your mood?

And what if I told you that you could do all of these things completely naturally?

Scientists used to think it was impossible. But new research reveals one common herb can produce all of these cognitive breakthroughs… and more.

Thousands of varieties—but only 1 scientifically verified to give you razor-sharp thinking

It's called Bluenesse®, a specialized variety of lemon balm (Melissa officinalis).

There are thousands of varieties of this herb. But there's only ONE that's scientifically verified to improve your memory, focus, word recall, and brainpower—and boost your overall cognitive strength.

In fact, it took scientists and farmers a year to identify and develop this particularly potent variety.

Bluenesse improves memory and increases focus and concentration by activating your brain's M1 receptors.

M1 sounds a bit like a Bond villain—but you can think of it like your "memory switch."

It's actually a very tiny, yet very powerful type of brain cell. M1s are in charge of a process called oscillation—which makes sure information flows freely between your brain cells.

Oscillation is a big deal. It's the only way you can store and retrieve your memories, learn new tasks, and stay focused.

If your M1s aren't activated properly, your brain—and specifically your working memory—feels sluggish. It's harder to remember things. Your focus seems fuzzy. And you don't seem to come up with answers or new ideas like you used to.

In essence, you have "senior moments."

But thanks to new in vitro research, we now know that Bluenesse can actually activate M1 receptors in the brain. And that helps the brain feel young again.

Now take a look at the effects in human clinical studies…

Sharper focus and revitalized working memory within ONE hour

In recent double-blind, placebo-controlled studies, 300 mg of Bluenesse was shown to:

- Improve memory and focus 13.5% compared to a placebo—in just ONE hour

- Improve math performance 38% in just three hours

- Dramatically boost working memory in just one hour. (Working memory is what helps you remember new "daily details," such as where you parked your car at the mall.)

- Boost alertness, even after three full hours. Take a look at this chart for more details.

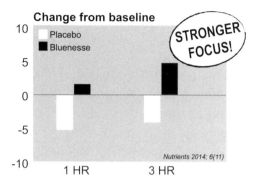

Change from baseline

STRONGER FOCUS!

Placebo
Bluenesse

Nutrients 2014; 6(11)

1 HR   3 HR

Can you imagine being able to feel your memory improve that quickly?

Rev up your recall abilities and stay cool, calm, and confident for hours

The Bluenesse groups also significantly outperformed the placebo groups in a test in which they saw 10 words for two seconds each, with a second in between each word. Immediately after all of the words flashed on the screen, the participants were asked to write down as many words as they could remember.

Then, 20 to 25 minutes later, they were asked to recall the words again. This tests long-term memory, or what I call "high-performance memory"—the ability to remember names, dates, places, and all of those security passcodes you have to create.

A refreshing "side effect"

In two human studies, the Bluenesse groups' memory and focus just kept improving. And their overall mental state improved as well. In fact, even three hours after taking Bluenesse, participants described themselves as "calm," "steady," "self-confident," and "comfortable."

There's quite a bit of research showing that lemon balm—and specifically Bluenesse—can help soothe stress away.

Lemon balm contains active ingredients that ensure your brain gets optimum amounts of GABA, an amino acid that helps you feel calm. And lemon balm is also known to contain compounds that help increase your levels of dopamine, the brain's feel-good chemical.

How to maximize your memory boost
with Bluenesse

Patients sometimes ask me, "When's the best time of day to take Bluenesse?" If you're not a morning person, you might want to take 300 mg as soon as you wake up. Think of it as a way to "activate" your brain, to get ready for anything the day has to throw at you. It can help you be bright and alert by the time you're ready to step out the door.

And if you need extra focus in the afternoon—for an important meeting, or a big project you're working on—it's OK to take it again. This "double-strength" dose (600 mg) has also been shown to have powerful effects on brainpower, while warding off fatigue and stress.

I'm so impressed by this "mental miracle," I actually worked with the manufacturer to bring Bluenesse to the U.S. I'm the first doctor in the country to use it, and others are beginning to follow my lead. The results in my patients have been phenomenal. They notice that they're able to think faster and more accurately. And they're thrilled to finally be free of those "senior moments" they'd resigned themselves to living with.

PART III

THE NEW HAMPTONS HEALTH MIRACLE

The next generation cure for diabetes, pre-diabetes, belly fat, metabolic syndrome, and so much more!

Chapter 19

10 Diabetes Myths That Could Kill You!

In this important chapter, you'll get an eye-opening look at just how shockingly INEFFECTIVE the mainstream's approach to diabetes really is. And I'm not just talking about drugs like Avandia or Actos. I'm talking about low-fat, doomsday diets… fake butter… and diet foods. You don't need them!

Let's get started…

MYTH #1
PREDIABETES ISN'T DANGEROUS

Let's get one thing straight. In many ways, pre-diabetes is MORE dangerous than diabetes.

It's dangerous because it's now an *official diagnosis*. Nowadays, when your doctor says you have "prediabetes," he immediately puts you on a drug to prevent the full-blown disease.

Plus, the American Diabetes Association's "new and improved" guidelines have lowered the blood sugar bar even further. This opened the door for millions of previously "healthy" people to start taking long-term heavy duty drugs.

In 2011, the prestigious *New England Journal of Medicine* published a study about the diabetes drug Actos. Researchers wanted to see if giving Actos to men and women with prediabetes would prevent them from developing the full-blown disease.

The study—conveniently sponsored by the drug's manufacturer—showed that men and women with prediabetes reduced their risk of developing the full-blown disease by a whopping 71 percent.

Predictably, all the major news outlets ran stories about the study.

But there's one small problem about Actos…it may increase your risk of bladder cancer. In fact, the FDA is currently investigating the link between Actos and bladder cancer. It appears that men and women who take it for more than a year increase their risk. Plus, it appears that the longer you take the drug and the higher the dosage, the greater your risk.

If this story sounds familiar to you, it should…

Remember Actos' ugly twin brother…Avandia? Actos and Avandia belong to similar class of drugs. Research showed that prediabetics who took Avandia also cut their risk of developing the full-blown disease. But Avandia appears to increase your heart attack risk. Now the use of the drug is strictly limited. Europe has banned it all together.

So what about metformin? This first-line diabetes drug hit the market in 1977. And, yes, it does appear to be safer than Actos or Avandia. Plus, studies show that it can reduce the progression to full-blown type-2 diabetes by 30 percent. But here's the bottom line…

Diet and exercise work better. *Far better.*

In fact, a recent study (again published in the *New England Journal of Medicine*) compared lifestyle changes to metformin in preventing type-2 diabetes.

The study followed more than 3,000 overweight men and women with elevated fasting and post-meal blood sugar levels. The researchers divided the men and women into two groups. One group took metformin for almost three years. The other group made changes to their diet and began exercising.

Three years later, the researchers checked back in on the patients. The metformin group reduced their diabetes risk by 31 percent (compared to a placebo). But the lifestyle change group *almost doubled* those results!

In fact, they reduced their incidence of developing type-2 diabetes by a whopping 58 percent!

So skip the scary drugs. You'll be better off in the long run.

With my NEW Hamptons Health Miracle, you can start to _safely_ drop those excess pounds and get your blood sugar in line…in just 6 weeks!

MYTH #2
EATING SUGAR DOESN'T CAUSE DIABETES

Simply put, you CANNOT develop type-2 diabetes if you do NOT eat sugar. Diabetes is a blood sugar disorder. Therefore, by eliminating sugar and anything that TURNS INTO sugar in the body, you eliminate your risk of becoming diabetic.

Think about it. How many people really gain weight from eating too much steak? You get full so quickly, it could never happen. But, combining it with sugar, or sugar-like substances and BINGO—you're on your way to getting diabetes.

On the other hand, I know plenty of skinny men and women who live on donuts and sweet tea. And guess what? They all come to me when they are diagnosed with diabetes or prediabetes, searching for answers.

Plus, a recent major study found that healthy men and women who consumed what government health experts consider "normal amounts" of high-fructose corn syrup experienced spikes in their cholesterol and triglycerides…within TWO WEEKS!

And high-fructose corn syrup…and we all know…is just another form of sugar. A deadly form, if you ask me.

For this study, 48 overweight but healthy adults began getting 25 percent of their daily calories from high-fructose corn syrup (HFCS). Remember, this amount is within current government guidelines for HFCS. But in just _two weeks_, their bad LDL cholesterol and triglycerides spiked through the roof.

You probably know sodas contain a ton of HFCS. But food manufacturers are sneaky. In many instances, you may not even realize your diet is filled with sugar! Always make sure to read food labels carefully. And even then, you have to be extra vigilant.

Take for example, my patient Jennifer. She came to me in her early 40s because she wanted to lose 20 pounds. *No matter what I try,* she said, *I gain weight. But I eat healthy, I don't understand it.*

Then I asked Jennifer to tell me about her typical meals. She said for breakfast she ate cereal with bananas or a plain bagel. A low-fat yogurt for lunch. And for dinner, some light pasta.

Jennifer's problem was very clear to me: She ate too much sugar and not ENOUGH fat. In fact, everything she ate either contained sugar or was itself sugar! No fat. Very little protein. And viola—she packed on 20 pounds.

Here's the truth about how your body works (no matter what the mainstream medicine might try to force feed down your throat)...

When you consume more carbohydrates that can be stored in your liver or muscles... and more than your brain needs to function... these carbs turn to GLUCOSE. The body stores three of these molecules together as a more efficient way of storing the excess energy.

This is called a triglyceride, and it explains why so many people with type-2 diabetes have high triglycerides.

These excess triglycerides are what clog up your arteries. That's why it's MORE dangerous to have high triglycerides than high cholesterol. High levels lead to higher incidences of heart disease and stroke.

To compound the problem, the ADA recommends that people with diabetes should start with consuming between 45 and 60 grams of carbohydrates per meal and make adjustments depending on how their blood sugar responds. PER MEAL?! That's more than I recommend *per day.*

Keep on their program for any amount of time and I'll bet you won't see your blood sugar budge.

Now, here's the good news...

On my program, you don't count carbs at all. Yes, that's right. All you have to do is stick to "slow release" carbohydrates like brown rice and

100 percent whole wheat, or better yet, grains like quinoa or buckwheat, and you're set.

MYTH #3
SKINNY PEOPLE DON'T GET DIABETES

I recently took the "DIABETES RISK TEST" on the American Diabetes Association's website. They asked me these six questions:

1. Age?
2. Does anyone in your immediate family have diabetes?
3. What's your ethnicity?
4. Height and weight?
5. Do you have high blood pressure?
6. Are you more active, less active, or as active as most men and women your age?

They ask *nothing* about sugar consumption or other symptoms. But these are FAR more important than your age, your family history, or even your weight! (As I said earlier...I've seen plenty of skinny sugar addicts walk into my office with full-blown diabetes.)

Plus, the ADA test is FAR too generous with your weight. A 160-pound woman who eats a donut every morning has a "low risk" of developing diabetes if she doesn't have a family history of the disease and says she's "more active" than her peers.

This is pure hogwash that lulls you into a false sense of security that relies on self-reporting, which is notoriously unreliable.

Here's a better list of questions to ask if you think you may be at risk to develop diabetes:

1. Do you eat sugar?
2. Do you eat processed foods?
3. Do you eat white flour?
4. Do you drink beer or wine?
5. Do you sometimes feel "cravings" for sweets or salty foods?
6. Do you sometimes skip your exercise routine?
7. Do feel light-headed or sleepy in the afternoon?

8. Do you ever feel depressed?
9. Do you weight at least 10 pounds more than you did in college?
10. Do drink diet soda?
11. Do you drink regular soda?
12. Do you cook with Canola oil?
13. Do you eat margarine?
14. Do you find it hard to lose weight, even when you exercise?
15. Do you have less energy than you did in your 20s?

If you answered yes to *ANY* of these questions, even if you're not overweight, it's a pretty good bet you're a candidate for prediabetes. But don't worry…more than half the country would fail my test, too.

Now, here's the difference. I WON'T put you on a drug or sawdust diet.

Instead, the answer is simple. By following my 6-week program, you'll feel (and look) better than ever! Plus, you'll silence your sweet tooth and supercharge your energy in the process.

MYTH #4
LOW-CAL & LOW-FAT DIETS
ARE YOUR ONLY OPTION

The grueling low-fat, calorie-counting "sawdust" diets just don't work. They don't work because they aren't satisfying.

Plus, when food manufacturers take out fat, they *add* in sugar and other nasty ingredients. In addition, low-fat diets can cause sharp DROPS in your good HDL cholesterol. They can also cause SPIKES in your triglycerides.

And worst of all, they don't contain enough *GOOD* fat.

Fat is extremely important to your body. It actually helps regulate your blood sugar. Fat takes longer for your body to digest. This prevents the sugar RUSH and lets sugar slooooowly drip into your bloodstream. Overall, it helps your metabolism operate much more efficiently.

Fat also plays a major role in the chemistry of your brain. Your brain is more than 60 percent fat and low-fat diets deprive your brain of essential fatty acids so vital to its function. That's why when you go on a sawdust diet you feel fuzzy-headed all the time or get the dieting "blues."

The American Heart Association diet recommends you limit total fat to less than 25-35 percent of your total calories. Although this diet has been shown to lower your total cholesterol, it lowers good cholesterol numbers and doesn't touch triglyceride levels. As I said earlier, this is a far more dangerous number.

Plus, low-fat diets may actually INCREASE your risk of diabetes.

A brand new study published in the *Annals of Internal Medicine* proves it.

In this clinical trial, researchers followed more than 3,700 adults ages 65 and over for three years. They asked the participants about what kinds of foods they ate.

Just as I would have expected...

Those who ate full-fat dairy products (we're talking delicacies you haven't dared to eat in YEARS, like heavy cream, and cheese) were actually 60 percent less likely to get diabetes than people who stuck to skim milk and reduced-fat dairy products.

Plus, they had:

- Less body fat
- Higher good HDL cholesterol
- Lower C-reactive proteinLower triglycerides

You see? This is what I've been trying to tell you! You need the fat.

But even my patient Irene had trouble accepting this new way of thinking. She came to me a few years back because she needed to lose 100 pounds. Plus, for the first time in her life, her blood pressure reading had started to creep up.

Irene had tried many low-fat, low-cal diets that made her track her points and calories. On these diets, she could eat as many carbs as she wanted, as long as she stayed within a certain amount of calories and fats for the day. But Irene found herself CONSTANTLY HUNGRY.

Sure, she'd lose weight for a time…but then pack the pounds back on.

Now, here's the good news about Irene…

Together, we got her off the sawdust dieting rollercoaster. She began eating a more balanced diet with MORE fat and SLOW-RELEASE carbs. In two weeks, she lost 15 pounds. In just 13 months, she lost all 100! Plus, her blood pressure came down to normal in just two months.

So throw out the low-fat yogurts and bring on the luscious, satisfying, and full-fat cream.

MYTH #5
ZERO CARBS = FASTER WEIGHT LOSS

On many popular diets, you must cut out ALL carbs during an induction phase. This requires you to go "cold turkey" off all carbs during the early phase of the diet. Don't even think about eating a grain of brown rice or a crumb of whole wheat bread. Heck, you can't even eat carrots.

Here's why my program filled with complex carbs works for the long-term…

Recent studies show that people who eat more complex carbs have a decreased risk of getting type-2 diabetes. In fact, complex carbs aren't the enemy. They help your body achieve a balanced state of insulin regulation. Plus, you need "slow carbs" for energy.

I'm not suggesting that you only eat slow carbs. Rather, strive to incorporate them into your balanced diet.

Slow carbs include: brown rice, oats, 100 percent whole wheat bread, barley, amaranth, buckwheat (kasha), kamut, teff, spelt, milo, millet, and quinoa. Vegetables also fall into this category.

Now, I know many of these may sound foreign to you but many of them are found easily at your local supermarket. Check the organic aisle first. If unavailable there, you can get them easily at your local health food store or you can have them delivered directly to your door by shopping online.

Whole grain cereals are usually the trickiest to pin down. So, here is a list of whole grain cereals you can safely enjoy on my decadent diabetes program:

- Cheerios
- Granola or muesli
- Nutri-Grain
- Shredded Wheat
- Wheat Germ
- Wheaties
- Wheatena
- Oatmeal made with steel-cut oats & no sugar

Avoid: Cream of Wheat, Cream of Rice, Grits, and other cereals marketed as whole grain that contain sugar.

You can also find whole grain pasta at your super market. You must check the food label. If it says "100 percent whole wheat," you're safe. You can also find pasta made from spelt, kamut, brown rice and quinoa.

MYTH #6
YOU SHOULD CUT OUT RED MEAT

Red meat is great source of lean protein and it will help regulate your blood sugar. Just make sure you choose lean cuts of organic, grass-fed beef. Yes, it's a little more expensive, but it's worth it. The meat tastes better...plus you won't have to worry about harmful hormones or pesticides.

Choose naturally lean cuts of meat, such as flank or sirloin. Marinate the steak for a few hours before grilling with lime juice, macadamia nut oil, and spices.

You'll also want to bring the meat to room temperature before grilling. This enhances the flavor.

Also, go ahead and leave the fat on the steak during grilling. After you take the steak off the grill, let it rest on the plate for 10 to 15 minutes. This allows the meat to reabsorb all the natural juices. Lastly, trim your steak before you serve it.

MYTH #7
YOU CAN'T DRINK ALCOHOL

According to recent studies, moderate drinkers (men who drank 5 to 6 drinks per week) are 20 percent less likely to die from all causes. Overall, moderate drinkers live longer than those who drink less.

Plus…

New studies show that alcohol can improve insulin resistance, lower triglycerides and LDL cholesterol, and increase HDL cholesterol.

Moderation is the key.

Men can indulge in up to four servings per week of distilled spirits. Women can enjoy up to two drinks per week.

MYTH #8
EGGS RAISE CHOLESTEROL & PACK ON THE POUNDS

Time and again, research has proved that eggs are not only safe to eat; they're good for you too! Eating them will even help you lose weight. Yet, this myth persists.

Here's the evidence to prove my point…

A 2007 study followed nearly 10,000 overweight but otherwise healthy men and women. The volunteers who ate one or more eggs a day *didn't* raise their triglycerides or cholesterol one iota.

Plus, they *didn't* raise their risk of heart disease or stroke. On the other hand, eating eggs seems to help raise GOOD cholesterol.

Plus, in a 2008 study published in the journal *Obesity*, researchers looked at breakfast habits of overweight men and women trying to lose weight. The folks who ate eggs in the morning lost more weight and felt more energetic than those who ate a bagel for breakfast. In fact, in an earlier study, volunteers who ate eggs instead of a bagel for breakfast lost 65 percent more weight!

MYTH #9
SKIP BREAKFAST TO LOSE WEIGHT

Skipping breakfast is one sure-fire way to sabotage your weight loss and your health.

Studies show that those who eat breakfast every day weigh less. So take a few extra minutes in the morning to make a nice omelet with a side of bacon (you can even throw in a slice of 100-percent whole wheat toast now and then, but try it without the toast the first few times—I bet you won't even miss it!) You'll feel great for the rest of the day. I guarantee it!

MYTH #10
MARGARINE IS BETTER THAN BUTTER

Walk through the grocery store dairy aisle and you'll see all kinds of "heart smart" margarine products. These products are nothing more than margarine with added plant sterols. Don't buy them.

Margarine is not better than butter…no matter how many vitamins or plant sterols you add. It is still fake butter and it contains trans-fatty acids even if it denies it on the label. The government allows products to be called trans fatty acid free if it contains less than 0.5 grams per serving. Yet, studies have shown that 3 grams per week can increase risk for heart disease.

Trans fats are bad news. They increase your risk of heart disease as much as some saturated fats do…if not MORE. Plus, they increase LDL (bad) cholesterol and decrease HDL (good) cholesterol. They also raise your lipoprotein(a) levels, impair arterial flexibility, and promote insulin resistance.

Yet somehow, the American public has been duped that their "heart smart" spread is safer than butter.

Chapter 20

Diabetes-Free in Just 6 WEEKS:

Your complete and exclusive, step-by-step guide to my NEW Hamptons Health Miracle

Ready to live diabetes-free? Then stop listening to what the diabetes industry has been telling everyone. I'm here with the best diabetes news in the last 30 YEARS.

Now YOU can indulge in the same healing secret sweeping the Hamptons. And discover for yourself just how easy it is…so much so, you'll soon be calling it, "a six-week vacation!"

In fact, you must start by forgetting the very idea of DIETING. This plan is simpler—and more decadent—than anything you've ever experienced.

Finally! All those useless years of deprivation are OVER…starting here and now!

Not since my mentor, the late Robert Atkins, M.D., has anyone had the guts to call the mainstream out on its deadly diabetes mistakes, or to offer a new cure. One so easy, and so enjoyable, it will completely transform the very course of diabetes care—and defeat your diabetes demons—for good!

I'm here to tell you that overcoming diabetes is not about pills, it's not about deprivation, and it's not about drugs.

You can indulge in loads of FABULOUS FORBIDDEN FOODS and help start to turn your blood markers around in JUST 6 WEEKS.

Did you know that most medical schools don't even require future doctors to study nutrition before they graduate? That means all the so-called diabetes experts out there probably have never learned the most basic way to treat diabetes: through smart eating!

I've spent my entire medical career studying nutrition and how it affects health, and that's how I know the anti-diabetes secrets that other doctors don't. The answers are not in a pill jar, on the surgical table, in the horribly misguided advice from the mainstream "diabetes experts," or in the latest fad diet.

The solution to diabetes is simple—and not only that, it's so sinful and so decadent…you'll think you're dreaming! All those so-called "diabetes experts" crowding the shelves and fighting for headlines have it all wrong.

Now YOU will know better than them. This easy, 6-week plan has worked miracles for my clients—and it will for you, too!

Just look at Joan, an A-list celebrity who had followed all the popular weight loss advice and was still 30 pounds overweight and diabetic. She came to my clinic not really believing that I could cure her—but she didn't know about my secret anti-diabetes weapon. I convinced her to follow my plan, and within three months she had lost 24 pounds.

Impressive, right? But even more impressive is the fact that her blood sugar readings were dramatically improved and she was able to cut her diabetes medications in half. In fact, at the end of six months she was off them altogether, her blood sugar was totally normal, and she was down 45 pounds!

And Joan isn't the only one. Ann, a famous clothing designer, was 56 when she realized she was turning into her mother—weight creeping up, blood pressure rising, and diabetes rearing its ugly head. Determined to stop the downward spiral, she came to me, and I put her on my plan.

The result? Her diabetes was stopped in its tracks, her cholesterol normalized, and her blood pressure was perfect—PLUS she lost 48 pounds!

This plan has had such dramatic effects for so many celebrities and A-listers that I can't in good conscience keep it a secret any longer. Others have paid dearly for the advice I'm about to give you for free!

So, if you're ready to feel better, look better, and live better…read on for the secret behind my NEW Hamptons Health Miracle and all the details of the 6-week plan!

The great diabetes myth

Diabetes. If it were a high school course, it wouldn't be science—it would be mythology. And unfortunately it's a Greek tragedy that's getting worse by the day. Far too many people suffer from this devastating illness, and worst of all, millions suffer without even knowing they have it.

Diabetes, and its precursor, blood sugar disorder, is a life-long, debilitating illness. It attacks the body from head to toe, robbing you of your memories, increasing your stroke risk, blinding you, rotting your teeth, clogging your arteries, ruining your love life—and the list goes on.

So there's the tragedy; now let's get to the mythology. Most people think diabetes starts when you get diagnosed. Not so. It starts at birth, and the fact is that most of us fall somewhere on the diabetes spectrum. Depending on your eating habits, genetics, and plain-old luck, it may develop into full-fledged diabetes or it may keep you treading water in the prediabetes zone. Either way, it keeps you from living the full and energized life you're meant to live!

Think of all the ways symptoms of diabetes shows up in your life, whether you're diagnosed with diabetes or not: That 3 o'clock energy plummet, forgetting why you went into a room, your caffeine addiction… you can thank blood sugar imbalance (a.k.a., prediabetes) for all these problems and more.

Isn't it time to fix it?

Of course, the first step to fixing your problem is admitting you have a problem. There are 25 million people with diabetes above the age of 20 in the United States and—even more surprisingly—an estimated 79 million Americans are considered to have prediabetes. Chances are you're one of them. I know I was.

But here's the good news. You can change it.

You can stop diabetes in its tracks and start living your life to the fullest—and all without deprivation, diets, or drugs! Read on for my simple, decadent, and life-changing plan.

Think you don't have to worry about diabetes? Think again.

Some people think they're safe from diabetes. They're wrong. Here are the top-5 misconceptions people have about why diabetes isn't a concern for them:

1. *I'm thin, so I don't have to worry about diabetes.* While it's true that obesity often goes hand-in-hand with diabetes, thin people are not immune. Even if you are of a normal weight, your risk factors increase if you are African American, Native American, or Hispanic; you eat a lot of sugar or refined carbohydrates; you don't exercise regularly; you have a family history of diabetes; or you are older than 45.

2. *I feel fine, so I can't have diabetes.* Diabetes doesn't always present with the classic symptoms (increased thirst, hunger, and urination, for example). In fact, most diabetics are diagnosed at a routine check-up.

3. *My doctor told me I don't have diabetes—just a "touch of sugar."* This is the most serious warning sign you can get. A fasting blood sugar reading of greater than 100 means you're at increased risk of heart disease and all sorts of vascular problems, including stroke. Stop what you're doing and start my plan for becoming **Diabetes-Free in Just 6 WEEKS** *today*.

4. *My doctor told me it doesn't matter how much sugar I eat.* This couldn't be further from the truth. Diabetes is a blood sugar disorder; therefore, by eliminating sugar and anything that turns into sugar in the body can significantly reduce your chances of becoming diabetic if you are predisposed to the disease.

5. *I've always been able to eat anything I've wanted.* Good for you. I hope you enjoyed it. Now it's time to step back and realize your body doesn't see it that way—at some point your body just can't compensate for all the wrong you have done. And with diabetes,

once the complications set in (which they do long before you even know you have the disease), it is really hard to make them go away. Now's the time to make a change.

Blood panel guarantee

If you follow this plan religiously for 6 weeks, I can virtually guarantee you'll see improvement in <u>every single measure</u> of health on your blood panel:

- Your LDL (bad cholesterol) will go down.

- Your HDL (good cholesterol) will go up.

- Triglycerides, C-reactive protein, homocysteine, fibrinogen, vitamin D levels, and total cholesterol will all stabilize.

And the most important marker of all—your blood glucose?

It will finally be on the road to normal!

Some other so-called experts promise results like these in just two weeks. You know the old adage "if it sounds too good to be true, it probably is"? That definitely applies here. You've spent years getting your blood sugar, cholesterol, triglycerides, and weight to the point they're at. Don't you think you'll need six weeks to get them back where you want them? But here's the thing—this plan is so SIMPLE, so SINFUL, and so DECADENT, that these six weeks will feel like a treat—not deprivation!

GET STARTED NOW: Six steps to my New Hamptons Health Miracle!

So you can see that the plan works—now are you ready to get to it? What follows is my sensible, easy, and indulgent plan for reversing your blood sugar problems in just six weeks.

You'll see there's nothing extreme about it—I'm not advocating a high-fat, ultra-low carb approach, or some expensive regimen that requires you to buy prepackaged meals from me. My approach is low in processed foods; high in good sources of protein; rich in vegetables, nuts, and low-sugar fruits; and rich in omega-9 monounsaturated fats. There's nothing gimmicky about it.

Follow these six principles for six weeks, and I can virtually guarantee that you will see every number on your blood panel improve. Your doctor won't believe his eyes!

Tap into your body's
HIDDEN FAT-BLASTING WEAPON

As rich and sinful as they seem, all the foods you'll read about in these special reports actually help your body tap into and maximize a little-known process, called TEF.

This secret process can help supercharge your metabolism, so that you burn more calories indulging in these "forbidden" foods than you would by eating so-called "diet" foods!

You see, as decadent as they are, all of the foods on my plan are minimally processed. And these types of foods make your body work harder to digest them, which kicks TEF into high gear, speeds up your metabolism—and makes you burn more calories.

And, based on my patients' experiences, adding macadamia nut oil to this program boosts weight loss even further.

1. Eat fish and eat other pure and lean protein.

Fish is great for the body, mostly because of its omega-3 fatty acids—especially DHA and EPA. These essential fats can lower triglycerides and raise HDL cholesterol—addressing two common problems for people with diabetes. Bonus: Omega-3s benefit the heart by reducing inflammation, decreasing the risk of clots, and preventing abnormal heart rhythms.

The downside of eating fish is the fact that pollution and poor fish farming practices have caused high mercury levels in fish. You can still reap the benefits without the risks by focusing on smaller fish like tilapia or sardines or taking fish oil capsules from a reputable source.

Stay away from top-of-the-food-chain fish like bluefish, striped bass, tilefish, swordfish, king mackerel, tuna steaks, and white and golden snapper, as well as any freshwater fish. When eating canned tuna, choose chunk light over solid white or albacore. This advice is especially important for women who are pregnant or nursing and those who plan to become pregnant within a year.

When eating fish, how you prepare it counts. Research shows that frying fish turns it from a wonder-food into a health-saboteur. Keep fish healthy by sauteing it in macadamia nut oil, baking it, or grilling it.

In addition to fish, I recommend other lean types of protein, including trimmed beef, trimmed pork, skinned chicken, and other animal forms of protein including eggs.

2. Eat nuts.

Our ancestors relied heavily on nuts in their diet, and it's little wonder why: Nuts are remarkably nutritious and were very easy to gather. We now know that they are not only full of protein, but they're also rich in important nutrients like vitamin E, folic acid, potassium, and magnesium. Plus, although they're high in fat, they're low in saturated fat and high in monounsaturated fat and omega-3 fatty acids. Important note: Peanuts are legumes, not nuts, and are therefore not included in this category.

3. Exclude trans-fatty acids.

If you want evidence of the failure of the food industry to promote health, look no further than trans-fatty acids. These aberrant concoctions are all over supermarket shelves for two reasons: They're cheap, and they increase shelf-life. Never mind the fact that they're killers. Trans-fatty acids, made when oil is hydrogenated, raise lipoprotein(a) levels, make arteries less flexible—raising blood pressure and stroke risk, promote insulin resistance, and increase the risk of diabetes. So basically everything you want to avoid if you're trying to live diabetes-free.

This is not one of those cases where moderation is the key to success— there is absolutely no safe amount of trans-fatty acid in the diet. In fact, as little as 2—3 grams of trans-fats per day can increase health risks. One single doughnut has 4 grams—and the standard American diet hovers somewhere around 40 grams a day. No wonder we're experiencing a diabetes epidemic in this country!

To avoid trans-fats, go immediately to your cupboard and look at every canned, bagged, or boxed food, and throw away anything that has the words "partially hydrogenated" or "vegetable shortening." First on your list should be margarine, the worst offender of all. Do what your grandma did: Use butter!

Another way trans-fats sneak into our diet is when we cook oils past the point where they produce smoke. Every oil has a different smoke point; olive oil smokes around 300 degrees F and therefore shouldn't be used for frying or sauteing. Macadamia nut oil has a smoke point of about 410 degrees F. This means you can cook with it without worrying about trans fats.

> ## Never Go Hungry
>
> Don't try to shortcut by forgoing food. Skipping meals can make you hungrier at the next meal, causing you to eat more than you should. Worse, hunger might tempt you to make bad choices when you do eat.
>
> ## Listen to Your Body
>
> • Eat only when you're hungry.
>
> • Don't go back for seconds.
>
> • Stop eating before you're full: It takes the brain about 20 minutes to realize your stomach is full, so give the two organs a chance to communicate!

4. Eat healthful fats: monounsaturated fats, specifically macadamia nut oil.

The high smoke point isn't macadamia nut oil's only health-boosting quality. In fact, when I discovered this oil, it completely changed my approach to healthful eating. I now use it every opportunity I get, and it's a big part of the success of my New Hamptons Health Miracle.

What makes macadamia nut oil so special? It's the fact that it's almost entirely composed of monounsaturated fats—85 percent, on average.

Plus, it's particularly rich in oleic acid, which increases the absorption of omega-3 fatty acids into the cell membrane, decreases total and LDL (bad) cholesterol levels, lowers triglyceride levels, and raises HDL (good) cholesterol levels.

When I tell you this plan will make you rich, this is the secret! Macadamia nut oil will make you monounsaturated rich—and provide health benefits that no amount of money can buy!

Other healthy monounsaturated fats include estate-bottled olive oil and avocado oil. Though they are best used at lower temperatures.

5. Eat your veggies (and some fruits)!

The produce section of your grocery store is a jackpot of antioxidants, micronutrients, and phytochemicals that rejuvenate the body.

You can't go wrong eating a colorful array of low-carbohydrate vegetables like greens, peppers, cucumbers, mushrooms, and bok choy. Starchy vegetables (peas, carrots, corn, potatoes, winter squash, beets, and so forth) are better left in the supermarket. There's a reason they feed corn to cows—to fatten them up!

Fruits make for a sweet and tasty treat, but some are a better choice than others when it comes to preventing and reversing diabetes. You'll want to focus on the ones that are lower in sugar, like these:

- Watermelon
- Honeydew
- Raspberries
- Cantaloupe
- Strawberries
- Blueberries

Stay away from fruit juices, which give you everything that's bad about fruit (sugar!) without the good stuff (fiber). And limit the sugary, tropical fruits like bananas, pineapples, mangoes, and papayas.

6. Consume moderate amounts of alcohol.

That's right, this plan allows for the occasional drink. Like I said, it's not about deprivation! Moderate amounts of alcohol (1.5 ounces of spirits four times per week for men, twice per week for women) actually benefit

Top-5 Age-Busting Foods

No one can argue with the blood sugar benefits of my New Hamptons Health Miracle, but what if I told you it can also make you look and feel younger?

People ask me all the time what I do to stay looking so young. Actually, it's quite simple: I follow the advice I've given you here, and I hardly ever deviate. What I've found is that the key to youthful, glowing skin begins in the stomach. The wrong food choices cause inflammation right down to the cellular level—and that inflammation leads directly to wrinkling, sagging, and premature aging.

These five favorite foods will take years off the reflection in the mirror—with the added benefit of being great for your whole body!

- Wild salmon: The pigment that makes wild salmon pink, astaxanthin, is a powerful foe of free radicals—those rogue molecules that damage cell membranes and DNA and cause skin to age. Farmed salmon, on the other hand, gets its pink color from manmade dye. Eating one serving of wild salmon every five days may prevent actinic keratoses—those ugly, brown, precancerous skin patches that become common with age.

- Leafy greens: Spinach, kale, and other leafy greens contain lutein, which protects the skin from sun-induced inflammation and wrinkles.

- Sweet potatoes: These contain beta-carotene, which balances the skin's pH, combats dryness, and promotes cell turnover—all resulting in smoother skin.

- Vitamin C–rich foods: Red and green peppers, broccoli, cauliflower, and of course, berries, cantaloupe, and citrus fruits, are all great sources of vitamin C—an essential nutrient for building collagen, the key component to younger-looking skin. These foods also contain bioflavanoids, which protect skin from UV rays and help prevent cell death.

- Lycopene-containing foods: Tomatoes (cooked), pink grapefruit, watermelon, and red peppers (cooked) are good sources of lycopene, a potent antioxidant that shields skin from sun damage from the inside.

Collagen isn't just important for skin health—it's also an essential part of the lining of blood vessels, helping them to expand and contract. So all the nutrients listed above can shave years off your heart and your complexion!

your health. Studies show the occasional drink actually improves insulin resistance and can prevent the onset of diabetes. Plus, people who drink in moderation—especially those with diabetes—decrease their risk for heart disease.

You'll notice I specified spirits and not wine, beer, wine coolers, or fruity cocktails. Why? Because distilled spirits like vodka are lower in carbohydrates, and your waistline will thank me.

What about exercise?

You're probably waiting for me to get to the part where I tell you to start jogging four times a week and lifting weights the other days. Well guess what—I'm not going to do that. You're about to overhaul the way you eat—for the better!—and that's enough of a change. If you don't exercise already, I advise that you don't start now. This plan is simple, decadent, and fun—it's not about pushing your limits and being uncomfortable!

Must-have nutrients to ensure your success

If you follow my New Hamptons Health Miracle without deviating for six weeks, you'll reach your goals. But let's face it—sometimes we could all use a little help getting to the finish line. Certain specific nutrients can boost your success and give you results faster than food alone. Think of them as a shortcut for faster results; these supplements will help you make up for damage done over the years and help you smooth over the bumps along the way. Recommended dosages are provided, but it's really up to the individual. If you take some of these together, you may get a synergistic effect and so may be able to take slightly less. Be sure to work with a doctor to monitor your blood sugar levels and adjust accordingly.

Benfotiamine (150-200 mg/day). This is a specialized, fat-soluble form of the B-vitamin thiamine. And one of its most notable benefits is its ability to interfere with the production of advanced glycation endproducts (AGEs). AGEs form in the body after prolonged exposure to excess blood sugar. And they destroy your tissues—quite literally aging you from the inside out. But benfotiamine helps prevent the formation of AGEs in the first place.

Mulberry leaf extract (200 mg/day). This herbal powerhouse supports blood sugar control in three ways. First, it helps your body process starch without impacting your blood sugar levels. It does this by distracting the enzymes in your intestine responsible for turning starch into sugar. These enzymes are "tricked" into thinking mulberry leaf extract is a sugar molecule and rush towards it. Meanwhile, starch is able to safely pass through your intestine without being turned into sugar. Second, mulberry leaf extract helps usher sugar from the blood stream into the cells that actually need it. In fact, a laboratory study reviewed in the *American Journal of Chinese Medicine* reveals:

Mulberry leaf extract could increase glucose uptake in cells by as much as 54 percent. And last but not least, mulberry leaf extract also helps your body reduce glucose production from within the liver.

Chromium (200 mcg, three times/day). Chromium is a trace mineral that most of us are lacking, largely because of nutrient depletion in farm soil. It is vital to blood sugar regulation, making it a great supplement for hypoglycemics, diabetics, and everyone in between. Another benefit: It curbs food cravings. Since it's exceedingly difficult to get this nutrient from food, I recommend taking it in supplement form.

Vanadyl Sulfate (25 mg): Used in Europe as a natural diabetes cure, vanadium sulfate mimics the effects of insulin in the body, allowing it to lower blood sugar and decrease insulin dependence. It does this by tackling one of the key elements of diabetes—insulin resistance.

Gymnema Sylvestre Leaf Extract (250 mg): This ancient Indian herb gradually lowers blood sugar, increases insulin, and cuts cholesterol and triglycerides—all very important exits off the road to diabetes.

Cinnamon extract (125 to 250 mg of Cinnulin PF® daily). This amazing standardized extract has singlehandedly revolutionized the cinnamon blood sugar market forever. Cinnamon's active ingredient is known as Type-A polymers. An in vitro study sponsored by the USDA showed that Type-A Polymers remarkably increased insulin activity 20 fold…which means blood sugar can be rushed to your cells like never before. In a 12-week randomized, placebo-controlled study, 250 mg of Cinnulin PF twice per day for 12 weeks was able to significantly improve

The new discovery that takes my Hamptons Diet to the next level

I've uncovered a new way to make my Hamptons Diet even better: Amino acids. You may already know they help build and repair nearly every cell in your body and keep the aging process in check. Now research out of the UK reveals they also help keep your heart healthy.

The researchers in this study collected data from 1,898 sets of female twins between the ages of 18 and 75. First they looked at the types of foods these women ate most frequently, and then measured the pressure, flow, and viscosity of their blood, and thickness of their arteries.

The results showed that women who had higher intakes of seven specific amino acids—arginine, cysteine, glutamic acid, glycine, histidine, leucine, and tyrosine—had significantly lower blood pressure compared to those with lower intakes of these amino acids.

In fact, women with the highest levels of these lowered their systolic blood pressure (the top number) by an average of 24.1 mmHg. Even a small reduction in systolic blood pressure—for instance, 5 mmHg—can potentially reduce the incidence of stroke, heart disease and an early death.

Researchers singled out five of the seven amino acids for helping to reduce hypertension: glutamic acid, arginine, glycine, cysteine, and histidine. These particular amino acids affect levels of nitric oxide, which helps dilate blood vessels, allowing blood to flow more freely. (Which, in turn, reduces blood pressure.)

Even better, evidence shows the remaining two amino acids in this group influence healthy blood sugar levels. In particular, leucine aids in insulin signaling, while cysteine helps with glucose uptake. And unbalanced blood sugar and diabetes go hand in hand with heart disease.

fasting blood-sugar levels. Plus, participants taking Cinnulin lost more body fat than those given placebo—and had healthier blood pressure.

Recent testing revealed Cinnulin PF has 4 times more Type-A polymers than three other cinnamon formulas on the market. And one of those formulas actually registered 0%! That's why I recommended Cinnulin PF over a generic extract.

Alpha Lipoic Acid (100-300 mg/day): Europeans have been using ALA for years to lower blood sugar levels and tackle another common complaint among diabetics—neuropathy. You can find ALA in foods such as red meat, organ meat, and brewer's yeast, or you can take it in supplement form.

Berberine (500 mg): Burn fat, lower blood sugar, and cholesterol and triglycerides with this ancient plant extract. Bonus: It just might make you less thirsty and, as a result, less chained to the bathroom.

Pycnogenol (50-100 mg): A diabetes cure in the bark of a tree? Researchers have discovered a wonder-nutrient in pine bark that lowers blood sugar, slows or prevents retinal diseases (common in diabetics), and improves blood flow.

Get started today!

See? I told you this would be easy! No gimmicks, no games, and NO DEPRIVATION. Mark the day on your calendar so you can look back six weeks from now and remember that this is the day that you chose to change your life and say goodbye to diabetes for good!

The Good Stuff

When choosing your foods, refer to this simple chart to sort the good from the bad.

	YES	NO
PROTEINS	Salmon, trout, sardines, flaxseeds, walnuts, lean meat, poultry without skin	Fried fish, untrimmed meats, too much bacon/sausage or milk
GRAINS	Whole grains like brown rice, spelt, quinoa, amaranth, wheat, and rye	White flour products, white rice, or any other refined or processed carbohydrates
VEGGIES	Salad-type veggies, including lettuce, spinach, kale, fennel, mushrooms, bok choy, celery, radishes, peppers, bean sprouts, and cucumbers	Starchy vegetables like peas, carrots, corn, white potatoes, winter squash, beets, parsnips, jicama, and plantains
FRUITS	Melons & berries	Tropical fruits
FATS	Macadamia nut oil; extra-virgin, estate-bottled olive oil; avocado oil	Hydrogenated oils and trans fats

Now go ahead…dig in, and get thin—
and beat your diabetes, for good!

Chapter 21

Diabetes Cheat Sheet for Even Faster Results:
Without eating less or lifting a finger!

My NEW Hamptons Health Miracle has sparked a national sensation, not only because it WORKS, but also because it's FUN!

This DECADENT crash course is so easy and so enjoyable; it will completely transform the very course of diabetes care. Follow my advice and you can:

- Escape the deadly diabetes snare
- Shed excess pounds to stay lean and sleek
- And look and feel fabulous at any age...

Yes! You can defeat your diabetes demons—for good! All you need are a few of my POWERFUL "secrets," FAST "tricks," and SIMPLE "short cuts" to supercharge your success.

GIVE IN TO YOUR CRAVINGS!

1. Go ahead...eat more chocolate!

Yes, eat more chocolate, the darker the better. You see, real cocoa contains powerful antioxidants, even stronger than those found in wine.

So indulge in more dark chocolate temptations. You'll lose weight and keep your blood sugar under control. Just skip the pre-made brownies or cookies. Make your own decadent treats, instead. They'll taste even better made with real cocoa and stevia.

Stevia is a natural sweetener that comes from a plant native to South America. There are many grades of it, so be careful when shopping. Unless you use a brand high in steviosides, there can be a bitter aftertaste.

Truvia™ is the newest form of stevia and you can find it just about everywhere. It actually contains a combination of stevia and erythritol, a sugar alcohol. But unlike other sugar alcohols, erythritol seems to cause fewer GI symptoms. But it's still a processed product, so use it sparingly.

In your baking, try to use straight stevia. Look for powdered versions in the sugar aisle of your grocery store. You can also find plain or flavored liquid stevia in health food stores or online. Plus, you can even find stevia-sweetened chocolate candies on the market nowadays.

I recommend making your own treats by melting 100% unsweetened dark chocolate. Mix it with 1-2 tablespoon of heavy cream and stevia. Drizzle it on berries or whipped cream for a decadent treat.

Also, here's a helpful stevia conversion:

6 packets of powdered stevia = ½ tsp stevia liquid = ¼ cup of sugar.

For more chocolate temptations, see my dessert recipes in Part 4…

2. Get a little tipsy!

I hope you enjoy and savor life. That's what's missing from most diets. They tell you how to CUT your cravings…CUT your calories…CUT your fat…and CUT the good things out of life!

But I say, "NO" to cutting!

You can enjoy life and indulge in a few naughty sins. Heck, even enjoy the occasional martini!

Yes, friends! You can (and should) enjoy moderate amounts of alcohol and still keep your blood sugar tightly under wraps. And don't worry; it won't make you gain weight either.

For women, you can have up to two glasses of distilled spirit drinks (1.5 oz of liquor) per week. Men can have up to four glasses of distilled spirit drinks each week.

Distilled spirits include rum, gin, vodka, tequila, and whisky.

My all-time favorite cocktail is an organic cucumber martini. Make it by mixing three parts organic cucumber vodka with one part dry vermouth. Shake and enjoy!

Now then, doesn't that make your Saturday nights a little more decadent?

3. Never skip meals!

Diets call for deprivation. But let me make this perfectly clear: Do NOT skip a meal and think you're on the fast-track to weight loss and blood sugar control. This will only make you hungrier and create metabolism problems. It also leads to overeating.

Instead, eat regular meals, spaced throughout the day. Strive to begin each meal with savory vegetable appetizers. Blanche veggies (lightly steam for 30 seconds or so, then run under cold water) and dip them in rich cream cheese, ranch dressing, peanut butter, or sour cream.

Also, if you must snack between meals, keep a bag of macadamia nuts or walnuts in your purse, car, or office drawer. This will help fend off cravings and dips in blood sugar.

4. Enjoy your carbs!

Carbs aren't the enemy! You just need to choose the right ones. In fact, carbs like 100 percent whole wheat, barley, quinoa, buckwheat, short-grain brown rice, and oats can actually help you lose weight and reign in your blood sugar. As do vegetables. Just remember corn and potatoes don't count. They are filled with too much starch.

Also, watch out for the hidden sugar in processed foods that contain whole grains. You'll find sugar hidden in whole grain breads, whole grain cereals, crackers, granola, and even in salad dressing.

Your safest bet is to avoid processed foods altogether.

5. Let those decadent desserts drive you wild!

Who says you can't enjoy your sweets? Decadent sweets. Rich sweets. Creamy sweets.

Have you ever tried making your own whipped cream at home? Once you try it, you'll never go back!

Make a berry float using 8 ounces of heavy whipping cream. This stuff is like heaven on Earth. Add to it 1 ounce of berries, 8 ounces of water, and ice. Combine all the ingredients in a blender. You can even add a packet of stevia to the mix. Then, pour into two parfait glasses and top with a few more berries.

Voila! Instant satisfaction. And you don't have to feel guilty about one biteful.

6. Keep your refrigerator stocked, not sparse!

It's pathetic. When you go on a diet, you eat the same thing day after day after day. And your pantry looks plain depressing with just "low-fat" cheese, yogurt, and turkey on the shelf.

I want you to take the COMPLETE OPPOSITE approach. Fill your refrigerator! Stock your pantry to the brim!

When you go shopping and see something fresh, buy plenty of it! You'll never feel deprived when your kitchen is stocked.

Plus, on most diets, entertaining goes out the window. Your friends won't stay friends for long if you serve them bland diet food. But try hosting a barbeque with Sticky Finger Spareribs, Sweet Potatoes, Dark & Decadent Fudge Brownies, and Cucumber Martinis on the menu! Now, that's what I call Hamptons-style entertaining.

7. Eat more fat to stay lean

When hunger strikes in the middle of the day (as it always does!), here's a fool-proof quick fix…eat a handful of nuts. They quickly fill your tank fast and keep you going until your next meal. This is because, unlike most snack foods, they contain protein, carbs, and fat.

Yes, nuts contain a lot of fat, but it's the good kind of fat. They are low in saturated fat and contain lots of monosaturated fat. So they will actually help you lose weight. In fact, a recent study followed 50 people with diabetes for one year. Half of the adults followed a low-fat diet. The other half followed a healthy diet that included a daily serving of walnuts.

Both groups lost weight in the first six months. But during the second half of the year, the low-fat dieters gained weight. On the other hand, the walnut eaters kept their weight off!

Plus, nuts are great for diabetics! Yale researchers recently found that diabetics who ate a handful of nuts each day for eight weeks improved their blood flow. And as you know, poor circulation is a major problem among diabetics. But eating nuts can help!

Enjoy macadamia nuts, walnuts, pecans, and hazelnuts. Eat them plain or roasted, not honey roasted. But skip the peanuts—they're not actually nuts at all, but legumes.

8. Get the waistline of a coffee-drinker without the jitters

Studies show that drinking coffee may help prevent the development of diabetes. In fact, Harvard researchers found that drinking four cups a day reduces your risk by almost 50 percent!

But that's a lot of coffee, even for a New Yorker like me. It's just too much caffeine.

Now, here's the good news…

You can get all the benefits of drinking coffee without the jitters. Try coffee bean extract. A recent lab test found that subjects given coffee bean extract reduced their visceral fat (belly fat) and body weight.

Researchers believe coffee bean works to block the absorption of fat and boost fat metabolism by the liver.

SHORTCUTS TO LOSE WEIGHT—FAST

9. Get an instant fix—now!

Okay. You're staring down a fresh box of donuts your colleague "kindly" brought to the office.

What do you do? *Take glutamine!*

It will INSTANTLY calm your sugar cravings. Pop a 500 mg capsule in your mouth when you feel a craving coming on. You can take up to 1,500 mg of it per day.

It's especially helpful early on in the program to help you keep you on track.

10. Drink water.

This is a cheap, surefire way to supercharge your weight loss. Studies show that when you're properly hydrated, you burn more calories—even when you're NOT exercising!

Plus, you'll save money.

The average six-pack of bottled soda costs upwards of $4 - $5. If you're like most folks and like to drink one or two of these a day, you'll save about $30 a month just from cutting out the soda! And while you're at it, skip the Crystal Light too. I have found that men and women who drink this lose weight much slower. Plus, for health reasons, you're better off without the aspartame.

How much water should you drink?

That's a great question! For quick weight-loss, divide your weight by 2.2. This is how much you weigh in kilograms. It's also how many ounces of water you should drink each day.

So, say you weigh 200 pounds. Divide that by 2.2 you get about 90. That's how many ounces of water you should drink each day to jump-start your weight loss.

11. Eat water too!

Here's one tasty trick you'll love to try. Certain foods contain high levels of water. So not only do they fill you up faster, they also help you lose weight.

Food	Percentage of water
Lettuce	95%
Zucchini	95%
Cucumbers	95%
Asparagus	90%
Broccoli	90%
Cauliflower	90%

Cabbage	90%
Spinach	90%
Clams	90%
Yogurt	85%
Cottage Cheese	80%
Eggs	75%
Brown rice	70%
Mozzarella Cheese	50%

Fill your plate with these foods to supercharge your weight loss.

12. Think green!

Green tea supercharges weight loss. It works by stimulating the breakdown of fat in your body.

It also improves kidney, liver, and pancreatic function.

You can drink green tea throughout the day, as I do. Or, you can take a green tea extract. Go for 300 mg three times a day.

13. Eat REAL food!

Your body knows the difference between real food and "diet" food. That's why diets fail. Your body wants you to take in real food.

So…

Always choose real butter over "heart-smart" plastic butter. Choose full-fat yogurt over fat-free varieties. Whip up mouth-watering omelets made with real eggs and cheese…not fake eggs and fat-free cheese—and always use the yolk. Make your own sinful desserts with real heavy whipping cream…not the fat-free white plastic filled with artificial ingredients.

I'd also skip the protein bars (they are nothing more than cleverly disguised candy bars) and protein shakes. These aren't satisfying. I could probably eat seven protein bars before feeling full. Instead, make Craveable Crab Quiche on Sunday and eat it all week for lunch along with a Ridiculously Delicious Raspberry Cheesecake Bar. Now that's what I call real food. (By the way, you'll find all of the recipes I've mentioned here—and many more—in Part IV of this book.)

14. Eat "high heat" foods

Here's another healthy way to trick your body into losing weight fast: Eat "high heat" foods. You see, not all calories are created equal. You body works much harder to digest foods with high thermic indexes.

Foods high in protein and fiber have high thermic indexes. That means they require a lot of energy to digest. On the other hand, high carb foods have low thermic indexes. They require very little energy to digest.

Strive to eat a fist-sized serving of protein with each meal. Also, eat lots (and I mean LOTS) of vegetables.

FILL IN THE GAPS

Taking vitamins is one of the best ways to get on the fast-track to optimum health and supercharge your weight loss. Plus, these key vitamins help protect you against the occasional slip up (everyone has them). But these nutrients will help fill in the gaps.

15. Daily Multivitamin

A good multivitamin will save you time and money. Plus, it's the basic building block to good health.

Now, I know that cheap grocery store brands will seem very tempting.

But skip them.

They're actually a waste of money and don't give you a fraction of what you need. Sure, they contain often 100 percent of the recommended daily allowance. But that's simply not enough. You'll save money and time by choosing a high-quality multi.

Take for instance, one popular brand on the market. The company claims that it is the No. 1 doctor-recommended brand (I certainly wouldn't want him or her as my doctor). But it only contains 60 mg of vitamin C. That's just pitiful. A good multi should contain almost 10 TIMES that much!

You see, unlike most mammals, we do not produce vitamin C on our own. But we need it badly. A potent antioxidant, it zaps free radicals that cause disease and premature aging.

Plus…

Vitamin C is critical to people with diabetes and prediabetes. As you know, most people with diabetes don't actually die of diabetes. They die of heart disease or stroke. But getting enough vitamin C may help reduce your risk of developing cardiovascular problems. You see, experts believe vitamin C helps to reduce oxidative stress, a major risk factor in cardiovascular diseases.

A study published in 2003 found that women who took vitamin C reduced their risk of fatal and nonfatal coronary heart disease. For this study, researchers followed 85,000 for 16 years. Two percent of the volunteers had diabetes.

After careful analysis, the researchers found that all of the volunteers who took at least 400 mg per day of vitamin C benefited. They were far less likely to suffer fatal heart attacks. Plus, they were far less likely to develop nonfatal coronary heart disease. This proved true even among the volunteers with diabetes.

But if you only take 60 mg of it a day you may be headed for trouble. You need at least 500 mg of vitamin C per day. Ideally, I'd like to see you get 1,000 mg, taken up to three times a day.

So yes, most store brands skimp on the good stuff.

You'll also want to skip any of the once-a-day brands. I know the convenience of an "all-in-one" pill is tempting. But it's simply not possible to fit all of the nutrients you need—in the quantities you should be getting—into one single capsule.

In fact, the very best way to get all the nutrients you need is to go powdered. Look for "scoop-able" vitamin formulas. You mix them with water and drink them. Your body will absorb more of the important nutrients when taken this way. And the manufacturers won't have to leave out any of the good stuff simply because it doesn't fit into a tiny capsule.

16. Vitamin D

After a good multivitamin, make sure to get plenty of vitamin D every day! It's the sunshine vitamin. Your body will make 10,000 IU of vitamin D after sitting out in the sun for just 30 minutes without sunscreen. I recommend you do this as much as you can, if you have the skin that can tolerate this exposure. But keep in mind that, if you live up North, the outdoors only works from May to September.

To help fill in the gaps, I also recommend taking a multi that contains 1,000 IU of vitamin D3. This is the form of vitamin D best absorbed by your body. You can get vitamin D alone, but you'll stretch your dollar by finding a multi that includes it.

Of course, that's easier said than done.

Let's take another look at the "doctor's No. 1" multivitamin. It contains 400 IU of vitamin D. And, yes, that's 100 percent of the RDA. But studies show that we need much, much more of this vitamin…especially if you are prone to blood sugar issues.

Just consider this…

A recent major analysis combined the results of 28 different studies involving almost 100,000 men and women. It showed that men and women who get the most vitamin D cut their diabetes risk by a **whopping 55 percent**!

 Plus, they reduced their risk of cardiovascular disease by 33 percent. And they cut their risk of developing metabolic syndrome by an impressive 51 percent.

You see, vitamin D seems to go to the root of the problem: your beta cells. These important cells produce insulin, the chemical that flushes sugar from your bloodstream.

But if you develop diabetes or prediabetes, your beta cells stop working. You stop producing insulin. Or, your body stops using it properly. As a result, sugar doesn't get to where you need it…to your cells and your muscles. It stays in your bloodstream instead. Hence, the term "high blood sugar."

Anastassios Pittas, M.D., an endocrinologist at Tufts University Medical Center, says that worn-out beta cells are "the main defect in type-2 diabetes."

But vitamin D may help recharge these "worn out" beta cells.

Dr. Pittas and his team recently recruited 92 pre-diabetic men and women. The volunteers all needed to lose a few pounds. Plus, they had above-normal blood sugar levels.

The researchers divided the volunteers into four groups. One group took 2,000 IU of vitamin D3 (cholecalciferol) once a day for four months. The second group took 400 mg twice daily of calcium carbonate for four months. The third group took both. And the fourth group took a placebo.

After four months, the vitamin D3 group significantly improved beta cell function. In fact, an expert estimated that beta cell function improved by 15 to 30 percent. Plus, the D3 group saw slight improvements in hemoglobin A1C, an indicator of blood-sugar levels over time.

So you see why getting enough vitamin D is important? Remember, look for a multi that contains 1,000 IU of D3. Your body absorbs this form best.

17. Essential Fatty Acids

After a good multi and some extra vitamin D, make sure you also add a high-quality fish oil supplement to your regimen. Fish oil contains important omega-3 fatty acids like EPA and DHA.

Studies have shown these nutrients are critically important to people with diabetes because they decrease your risk of cardiovascular disease. Remember, most people with diabetes die of a stroke or heart attack... not high blood sugar. So here's what omega-3s can do to help:

1. Prevent arrhythmias that can lead to sudden death.
2. Decrease your risk of developing harmful clots that can lead to heart attack or stroke.

3. Prevent the development of atherosclerosis.
4. Improve elasticity of your blood vessels.
5. Help to lower blood pressure.
6. Squash inflammation through the body.

And that's not all…

High triglycerides are a common problem among people with diabetes and prediabetes. These harmful blood fats can get out of control when you eat too many simple carbs.

But taking fish oil can help here, too.

A recent meta-analysis looked at the results from 18 different clinical trials. Researchers found that men and women with diabetes who took fish oil supplements lowered their triglycerides by 31 mg/dl compared to placebo.

Plus…

In 2006, scientists reviewed numerous clinical trials involving EPA and DHA. They found that taking fish oil reduces your risk of all-cause mortality as well as your risk of suffering a fatal heart attack. So not only does fish oil appear to improve your heart health… it seems to protect you against *all* types of early death.

Now, most western diets contain far too many omega-6 fatty acids (found in vegetable oils) and not enough omega-3 fatty acids.

But taking a fish oil supplement will help to correct this imbalance. Look for a capsule that contains EPA and DHA. You want the total daily dosage to reach 3,000 mg.

Sure, I know a lot of people cringe when I tell them to take fish oil. But here's the key: Take it with meals! You'll have far fewer fish burps. I usually swallow mine about mid-way through my meal to minimize the fish aftertaste.

Also, you want to make sure you get your fish oil from a reputable company. Many brands on the market contain contaminants and mercury. These toxins accumulate in fish. So it's important to find a brand that only contains highly-refined fish oil.

18. Chromium

No diabetes program is complete without chromium. Sure, it's an old standby, but it's also a MUST for people with diabetes and prediabetes.

Here's why…

Chromium helps your body use insulin more efficiently. It also "turns on" insulin receptors in your pancreas. It helps transport sugar from your blood to your cells, where you need it! Lastly, it helps regulate how your body digests fat.

In recent studies, chromium reduced blood sugar among type-2 diabetics. It even reduced the need for insulin.

Chromium is an essential trace mineral once found in our soil. So 100 years ago, simply eating vegetables from the garden gave you enough of this important mineral. Not today.

Poor farming practices have depleted our soils. That's why studies show that as many as 90 percent of Americans don't get enough chromium! Plus, as you age, your chromium levels decline.

The only *real* answer is to take it daily as a supplement.

Look for a supplement that contains at least 200 mcg of chromium. According to a study recently published in the *Journal of the American College of Nutrition*, this is how much diabetics or prediabetics should aim to get each day. It's also the amount used in many clinical trials shown to lower blood sugar. But you'll have to look hard for a multi that contains this much chromium. Most fall waaaay short. Let's again look at your typical daily multivitamin. It contains an absurdly low amount of chromium. Just 35 mcg.

So, again, choose your multi wisely!

19. Pycnogenol—one of the most important powerhouses you've never heard of!

This one little-known, all-natural discovery will revolutionize your health. It's a MUST for EVERYONE with blood sugar issues, high blood pressure, or poor circulation. But you've probably never heard of it. Even among nutritional gurus, it's discussed very little. And that's a shame, for several reasons…

First off, Pycnogenol helps to improve blood flow throughout your body. It does this by supporting the health not only of your veins and arteries but also of all the small blood vessels and capillaries that deliver oxygen-rich blood to every part of your body—from your fingertips to your pinky toe.

You see, Pycnogenol produces and maintains collagen and elastin throughout your body. Yes, these two proteins help you maintain a youthful appearance. But what you probably don't know is that they're essential to your veins and arteries as well! In fact, your veins and arteries are built out of collagen and elastin.

That's how Pycnogenol revives your worn-out circulatory system. Plus, it goes to work fast!

Just consider this…

Italian researchers recently followed type-2 diabetics with muscle cramps and poor circulation. They divided the patients into two groups. One group received 200 mg a day of pycnogenol for four weeks. The other group got a placebo.

The placebo group didn't get any better. But in just four weeks, the pycnogenol group significantly improved their blood flow! They also experienced fewer cramps and less muscle pain. Even patients with intermittent claudication felt better after just four weeks of taking Pycnogenol.

Plus, Pycnogenol helps to lower blood sugar.

In another recent study, researchers gave people with diabetes either 100 mg of Pycnogenol or a placebo for 12 weeks. The Pycnogenol group significantly lowered their blood sugar levels compared to the placebo group. Plus, they lowered their glycated hemoglobin levels (or

HbA1(c) levels). This is another tool doctors use to evaluate diabetes.

Pycnogenol works by regulating the release of glucose into your bloodstream. In a recent study, scientists found that Pycnogenol significantly delayed the uptake of glucose after a meal. In fact, it delayed glucose uptake 190 times more than a commonly-prescribed diabetes medication.

Lastly, Pycnogenol helps support healthy blood pressure. In another recent study, researchers gave 125 mg of Pycnogenol to type-2 diabetics with high blood pressure. After just 12 weeks, 58 percent of the diabetics lowered their blood pressure so dramatically…they were able to cut their meds by half! Plus, they significantly lowered their fasting blood sugar levels as well as their LDL cholesterol.

I recommend taking 100 mg of Pycnogenol per day if you're prone to blood sugar issues. This is the dose used in more than 200 clinical research trials.

20. Natural extract works as well as metformin!

Over and over, you hear about the benefits of taking cinnamon. But one natural agent called berberine blows cinnamon out of the water.

In two recent studies, researchers divided newly-diagnosed diabetics into two groups. One group took berberine and the other group took metformin.

Shockingly, berberine performed just as well as—if not BETTER than—metformin! Makes you wonder why endocrinologists hand out metformin at all, doesn't it?

Here's how the data broke out at the end of three months. The berberine group:

- Lowered fasting blood sugars from 191 to 124 ml/dL
- Cut post-prandial blood sugar (blood sugar after eating) from 356 to 199 mg/dL

For more on berberine, see page 48.

Chapter 22

Decadent Dining Out Plan:

How to eat out every day,
still lose weight, AND defeat diabetes

Love to dine out? Of course you do!

And so do my Hamptons clientele of course, which is why I've spent so much time designing a program that could fit easily into the busiest lifestyles.

In fact, being able to still "hang out" and "be seen" is probably the No. 1 request I get when working with new clients.

Take Chuck for example. He was 47 when he first came to see me. He was 50 pounds overweight and had high cholesterol. He was an investment banker that worked long hours and traveled the globe. And he loved every high-strung minute of it.

But he was also on the road to diabetes, and a heart attack waiting to happen. And he knew it.

Clearly, Chuck needed a diet that would conform to his lifestyle. There was no way I could put him on a plan that required him to cook at home, or that would make him look foolish when he was dining out with clients.

He needed a program that would give him all the benefits of "dieting" without looking like he was on a diet!

Then there's Brady.

A Wall Street trader, used to the perks that come along with that position— fancy clothes, fancy beach houses, and lots of wining and dining. He also needed something that would work with his lifestyle.

Fortunately, The New Hamptons Health Miracle fits them to a "T"!

My program is easy to follow, whether you're cooking at home, eating out, or even traveling around the globe

And with just a few simple tricks, eating out will be even more enjoyable than before—guaranteed!

Imagine…NO MORE side-salads with dressing on the side for your main course…NO MORE turkey burgers sans mayo, cheese, or bacon…and NO MORE "no thank you" for dessert!

Instead, now you can go ahead and order that T-Bone with mushrooms and onions with creamed spinach on the side, or grilled salmon with broccoli and a sweet potato, or a juicy rare burger with bacon and cheddar, and follow it all up with a big bowl of berries in rich, heavy cream.

Just a few simple special requests and modifications to the items you see on the menu is all it takes.

And I'm here to tell you—don't be afraid to do this!

It's common practice nowadays, and most places are happy to accommodate you. And, if they're not, why would you want to eat there anyway? (After all, isn't the customer always right?)

And I can tell you this…if a restaurant wouldn't agree to make a few small changes to Chuck or Brady's orders, no matter where they are eating, they wouldn't tolerate it. And you shouldn't either! Simply move on to one that will.

And this advice doesn't just apply to eating out

When you make dinner plans with friends, explain that you're doing your best to stick to a healthy diet, and ask if you can pick the restaurant—and choose somewhere you know you can find (or special order) something nutritious.

When you accept an invitation to dine at a friend's house, go ahead and ask what's being served… and offer to bring a side dish. (And make sure it's healthy! You don't have to advertise this fact, but you'll have some peace of mind knowing that you can eat it—plus, you're doing all the other guests a favor, too!)

And if the main course isn't something you feel comfortable eating, just explain your situation to the host or hostess and ask if they would mind if you brought a grilled steak with you. Good friends will understand, and be glad to support you. And in fact, they may actually ask for a bite of whatever you bring later!

And that's really what I'm getting at here...

The road to good health can't be paved alone

Don't be afraid to be vulnerable and ask for help. Others can't support you if they don't know what to do.

If you let people know what you need, you'll be surprised at how much easier it is to achieve your goals.

Now on to the good stuff...

Following are a few tips and tricks that you can follow when dining out.

They'll work whether you're hitting the local drive-thru, diner, or a high-end, 5-star restaurant.

1. Focus on the core foods from my MUST LIST first—to narrow your options.

Remember, there's really not much you need to know to put my plan for defeating diabetes into action, especially when it comes to which foods to enjoy and which to avoid. I really tried to make it as simple as possible, so you don't have to pull out any complicated point guides, food diaries, or calorie counters.

When it comes to making a choice from the menu, depending on where you go, it can quickly become overwhelming. After all, some menus are a half a dozen pages long! Really?! You may want to avoid the temptation of such establishments from the start. But if you must...

Start by focusing on options for your main course first, and narrow down the possibilities by identifying those dishes that feature foods from the following MUST list:

Main Course Musts:
- Beef
- Poultry
- Pork
- Fish
- Seafood
- Eggs

> **QUICK TIP:** *Be sure to check out the Dinner Entrée section— even for breakfast and lunch, just check with the server that they can prepare anything at any time. You may also find some surprisingly good options in some Appetizer sections as well.*

2. Narrow it down to how the main course is prepared.

- Stick with the following cooking methods: grilled, broiled, baked, or steamed. Which shouldn't be too hard, especially if you have the flexibility of choosing from the Dinner Entrées. And if you're doing sushi, stick with the hand rolls without rice or sashimi (which is the raw pieces of fish without the rice). And soy sauce is ok, by the way.

- Avoid anything breaded: While you may be able to make a healthy breading for dishes at home, in most cases, what you'll find in restaurants is not a healthy option!

- Avoid anything fried: Unless you find a rare gem of a place that uses macadamia nut oil to do it!

- Avoid sandwiches/buns if you can. If you can't see below.

3. Consider minor modifications to the Main Course item—beware the bun, sauces, and condiments!

Ok, so up until this point, it should be pretty straight-forward, and fairly easy to narrow down your choices. But this may be one of the trickier steps. And it's definitely one of the most important.

First, the more obvious—avoid the bun. Simple. Meats sit on a plate quite nicely…no need to hide it under a bun, no matter what the bun's made of!

Second, if you must order a sandwich and just can't stand to the contents sitting out naked on the plate, ask to have it set on a bed of lettuce instead. And if that simply won't work for your ham & cheese, ask to swap out the sandwich bread with a tortilla wrap instead. These days, you'd be hard pressed to find a restaurant that doesn't offer something in a wrap. This means they must have them in the back. Why limit the wrap option to just the item already on the menu?

Again, don't be afraid to ask...you may end up starting a new trend!

And finally, skip the sauce and the condiments! You'd probably be shocked to find out just how much sugar is hiding in those toppers. But for someone with diabetes, they can be your worst nightmare... just a little too much, and they can sneak up on you out of nowhere and throw your blood sugar out of whack so fast, you won't have any idea where it came from!

Catsup contains more sugar than ice cream, so stick to whole-grain mustard or just a dab of mayonnaise (just NOT the fat-free versions, please—they also contain more sugar than the regular versions).

And as for the sauce, unless it's Hollandaise or something made with heavy cream...skip it. Or, better yet, see if they have some blue cheese or feta to sprinkle on top, or have them melt some cheddar or sauté some onions or mushrooms for you, and just some fresh lemon or melted butter (not margarine), on the side for fish is all you need. Or ask if they have a bit of soy sauce in the back that you could get on the side.

> *QUICK TIP: While the server goes around to ask everyone with pasta if they'd like fresh parmesan on top—go ahead and ask to have some grated on top of your meat! Do the same with the fresh-ground pepper as well...many restaurants will offer it to patrons with salads...and there's nothing like a bit of fresh cracked ground pepper on a grilled chicken breast or grilled steak.*

4. Switch out your sides.

Unfortunately, these days, it's next to impossible to find an entrée on a menu that doesn't come with some sort of starch or pasta on the side...French fries, potatoes, potato salad, potato chips, pasta salad, and even sides of spaghetti!

Fortunately, these days most restaurants are used to swapping out sides for the low-carbers and low-fatters alike. Really EVERYONE should be swapping them out just for the sake of it being a healthier option regardless of what "diet" you may be following.

Stick with veggies or a side salad. Just remember, corn is not a vegetable, it's a starch, and just like potatoes, it's not a healthy option! Green is always best.

And if they have them, and you can't do without a starch, substitute a baked sweet potato if you can—just be sure they don't load it up with cinnamon sugar—a little butter and plain cinnamon on top is just delicious!

Another option for when they're in season, or if you're lucky enough to live or vacation where it's warm...is a side of mixed berries.

5. You can always opt for a salad.

If you've gone through all the steps above and just aren't finding something you'd like—or if the dinner entrée menu isn't an option at lunch—you can always count on finding a salad. Just keep the following in mind:

- mixed greens and romaine are always better than iceberg

- make sure the meat or seafood you add is grilled, not fried

- skip the dressing and just ask for some fresh ground pepper, sea salt if they have it, and maybe a little high-quality olive oil and a slice of lemon on the side

- antipasto is always a safe bet and even salad nicoise if they have it (a French salad made with a mixture of fresh vegetables and usually tuna and anchovies)

6. Go ahead and consider the apps…

Appetizers that is. (I promise, my program is not so complicated that you need some fancy phone app to keep track of everything!)

Once you decide on your main course, you may actually feel that what you've chosen will be filling enough. Which is why you should always start by deciding on the main course first. You will typically find healthier options in the entrée section compared to the Apps, and ultimately more satisfying as well.

But if you really feel the need to pick at something first, you can always start with a small salad. Or ask your companions to consider something on the healthier side.

All you need to do is apply the same rules as above to zero in on your selection.

7. Go ahead and consider dessert…

Just be prepared to get creative. Unfortunately, while it's quite easy to whip up a healthy and still decadent desert at home…it's tough to find a restaurant that doesn't have something laced with sugar.

If you find a dark chocolate truffle or something of the like, you may be in luck. Just double-check with the waiter to check with the chef to see if they've added sugar. If you really want chocolate, you can see if any of their chocolate desserts are topped with a dark chocolate bar. If so, just ask if you can get just the bar!

Another option is to look for berries and cream on the menu. Again, you may have to get creative. Just because they don't have it listed in the dessert section, doesn't mean they can't put it together for you. If they have a fruit salad side or berry garnish on something else, and heavy cream for Alfredo or for making fresh whipped cream, they might put it together for you.

If you're lucky enough to splurge on a 5-Star restaurant for some special occasion, another great option for dessert is actually a cheese plate!

And finally, you can always just top the night off with a hot cup of coffee with a splash of heavy cream, a steaming cup of green tea, or my favorite, an ice-cold martini.

8. Take your time!

If you're not hitting the drive thru and actually have the luxury of some time to sit and enjoy your meal…please, take your time and enjoy it! When you're relaxed and take the time to chew your food fully, savor the flavors, and enjoy conversation between bites…you'll give your body a chance to feel satisfied sooner, and you may actually eat less.

Unfortunately, many servers feel pressured to turn over the tables quickly—meaning they hardly give you time to sit down and open the menu before they're in your face demanding an order.

So when they come to ask what drink you'd like to start with, order your water or cocktail and go ahead and give the waiter a heads up from the start that you would like to sit for a bit and take your time… so no need to hurry. You may be surprised to find they appreciate it!

9. How to "fake it" in style

Ok, ok…I'll admit, all the substitutions and modifications can seem a bit "high maintenance." But remember, you're saving your life here…isn't a little extra attention to the details worth it? And after a while, this will become second nature and it won't seem so "odd" at all. In fact, you will start to find it strange when others don't eat like you.

If you're concerned about being a burden on the waiter or kitchen, simply offer to leave the tip and provide a little more than the typical 15-20%. They'll love to see you and make any accommodations next time you're in. Or, if they make you feel uncomfortable, like I said earlier, go somewhere else next time!

If you're not dining with friends and family who are supporting your efforts, but rather important potential clients, or even your boss, here are a few quick tips:

• Go ahead and ask for the dressing or sauce and condiments on the side (everyone does that these days anyway).

- Asking for an additional side of sautéed mushrooms and onions or feta cheese or blue cheese is also usually socially acceptable in most restaurants. Certainly if you go to a steak house.

- Get the bun or the bread, then remove the meat from it, and eat it with your fork and knife. Usually once the food is served, everyone's so absorbed with their own eating, they don't notice exactly how you're eating your own food! And the servers clear plates so fast these days, they may not even notice a full bun left on the plate…if they do, just say you weren't feeling as hungry today.

- Go ahead and substitute the side for veggies or a salad—again, this is very common practice these days, and would probably be admired. If for some reason you can't substitute, go ahead and order an additional side salad and just eat that. Leave the rest on the plate with your bread. Again, chances are, no one will notice if you don't take a bite.

Chapter 23

Amazing Hamburger Cure:

How I cured my own obesity for life, with the help of America's favorite "junk food"

I'd like to let you in on a little secret…something you'd never suspect just looking at me. But it's something I share with all my new patients when I start them on my program, I tell them:

"I know you can do this—because I did."

That's right: My experience with weight loss began long before I ever became the "doctor to the stars."

You see, I grew up in what I consider a very normal Italian-American family. Loving, close-knit and completely obsessed with food. We ate pasta and bread with every meal, *and we ate all the time.*

Needless to say, we were all overweight—my parents, my two older sisters and me. But that was the norm in my family, so I never thought much about it, until I hit high school and…

By the time I was 15 years old, I was a whopping 240 pounds, plagued with asthma and allergies, and the brunt of many cruel jokes amongst my peers.

I knew I had to do something.

Then it hit me: As much as I loved and respected my parents, *I was in charge* of what I put in my body.

And simply by choosing different foods, I could change the way I looked. (As it turned out, I would also completely revitalize my health…but at 15, I was mostly concerned with appearance!)

So I started that very day.

Six weeks later I'd lost 60 pounds. Then, believe it or not, I managed to keep it off and stay healthy…

BY EATING HAMBURGERS!

Well, it proved so successful for me, that now I'd like to share this little secret with you.

Mind you, this is definitely not something I would recommend anyone follow for a long period of time. But, if you're a lover of hamburgers, then this is a nice little trick to kick-start your efforts for a few days!

And if you follow it longer than that, please be sure you are also taking a high-quality multivitamin, a fish oil supplement, and something for added antioxidant support, since you won't be getting everything you would normally get from a greater variety of meat, fish, and vegetables in your diet. But, when you consider this trick from a logical perspective… it can make starting your new dietary efforts easier than ever. It takes all the stressful guesswork out of what your next meal will be—and definitely makes grocery shopping a snap.

Plus, when you do it alongside my *3-Day Sugar Cure*—each meal will leave you fully satisfied and your sugar-levels steady as a rock, which will make getting through those first three days a cinch. And help rocket you to your blood sugar and blood panel goals even faster than you thought possible.

So what exactly did I do? Remember, I was only 15, so it wasn't all that complicated…

I simply ate a hamburger at each meal, made with lean ground beef—without the bun, with a salad of mixed greens sprinkled with olive oil for dressing.

No snacks in between. And water to drink.

Of course, I didn't know about the value of macadamia nut oil then, like I know now. So I would definitely switch that for the olive oil.

As for the size of your burger, it depends on your appetite. A quarter pound burger should really be plenty for everyone. But if you need a little extra, go for it. Just be sure to eat slow and allow time for your body to process what you're putting into it and realize that you're actually starting to get full. I would bet you won't need as much as you may think to fill it.

And if a quarter pound even seems too much for you, try making up a batch of smaller sliders—these would be great for breakfast, and you can make them up in a larger batch and keep them in the fridge to warm up when you're ready.

It's that simple.

Of course, now that I'm older and actually know how to cook…I would probably have mixed it up a bit to make it more enjoyable.

Try topping your burger or, for a more gourmet delight, mix the different cheeses inside the burger—cheddar, provolone, pepper jack, or even jalapeno cheese. You can also mix it up with sautéed mushrooms, onions, peppers or of course bacon.

As for the salad, you can mix that up as well—try romaine, spinach, or even an arugula salad. And sprinkle some macadamia nuts or even blueberries on top.

I know that once you decide, like I did, that you're ready for a change… you'll quickly discover how getting thin—and ditching diabetes for good—is almost TOO EASY with my NEW Hamptons Health Miracle. It's so SIMPLE, and so ENJOYABLE, it just makes PERFECT SENSE.

Chapter 24

3-Day Sugar Cure:
Start reversing diabetes in just 72 Hours

When it comes to pinpointing the cause of diabetes and all its complications, it essentially boils down to ONE thing.

And despite what the American Diabetes Association would have you believe, it's NOT FAT, and it's certainly not cholesterol.

It's *SUGAR*.

Simply put, it's highly unlikely that you'll develop type-2 diabetes if you do NOT eat sugar—at least not a ton of it. Diabetes is a blood sugar disorder. Therefore, by eliminating sugar and anything that TURNS INTO sugar in the body, you eliminate your risk of becoming diabetic.

And if you have diabetes, kicking your sugar cravings is the fastest thing you can do to get you on the road to reversing your diabetes for good!

Think you can't live without sugar? Well I think you can.

In fact, I know you can. And I've helped hundreds of others do it… starting with this one simple technique.

All it takes is 72 hours. That's it.

Imagine, 72 hours from now, you'll be well on your wait to living diabetes-free for the rest of your life.

So isn't it worth a shot?

I've seen even the most diehard sugar addicts succeed.

Just remember to take it day by day. Don't try to make all your changes at once, keep it easy. Make one change at a time, and in just 72 hours you'll be reformed—for good!

Ready to get started?

Day 1: Cut the Crud

This first day is simple: Just avoid everything that you know has sugar without even having to think about it. Cookies, cakes, ice cream, soda—toss them all.

If it seems like just one small sweet won't hurt you, try looking at the sweet and visualizing all the sugar it contains. An ounce of hard candy? Picture a 5-teaspoon mound of sugar! A slice of cherry pie? Make that 10 teaspoons.

Now imagine sitting down and eating that mound of sugar, and you'll see just how damaging those sweets really are!

Day 2: Unrefine Your Diet

Get rid of all the processed, refined, and simple carbohydrates in your diet. This means white rice, white flour, sugar, corn syrup, and fruit juice (did you know apple juice has more grams of sugar than a fully leaded soda?).

Whole grains (quinoa, brown rice, and millet, for example) are A-OK.

Day 3: A Sugar by Any Other Name

So you switched to whole wheat bread. Great! But did you read the label to make sure it didn't have any simple sugars? You should—and don't just trust the marketing claims, such as "no sugar added."

It's surprising how many seemingly safe foods hide sugar, corn syrup, and refined carbohydrates. Take a close look at the ingredients list and avoid sugar, obviously, but also these ingredients:

- Honey
- Barley malt
- Rice syrup
- Fructose
- Concentrated fruit juice
- Maple syrup
- Cane sugar
- Anything that ends in —ose or —ol

Now here's the part where I get the most raised eyebrows, but hear me out: I need you to give up fruit on day three. Fruit is largely sugar (did you know a banana has 6 grams of sugar?) and therefore needs to be included in the sugar-elimination challenge.

This isn't forever—just until your metabolic imbalances have been corrected, at which point you can add low-sugar fruits like melons and berries back in.

You Did It!

You should be extremely proud of yourself.

If you were as sugar addicted as most Americans, it was probably a tough three days. Sugar is everywhere! We can't escape it; it's in every office, at every social gathering. But this challenge showed you that you can do it, even if it's sometimes a bit difficult.

And now that you're through the first three days, you've made it past the hardest part. So even if you don't feel great just yet, you will—as long as you continue to stick with it. Your body has begun to readjust

---

Sweet Drinks

One of the hardest things for some people to give up is sweet drinks—and on this plan, soda has got to go. (Yes, that includes diet soda!) But that doesn't mean you need to stick to plain old water. One of my favorite ways to make water more satisfying is to infuse it with flavors I love. I keep a pitcher of this infused water in my fridge for when I need something more interesting than water—the cucumber makes it crisp and refreshing, and the mint satisfies my sweet tooth.

Ingredients

½ gallon filtered water

1 small cucumber, sliced thin

½ cup fresh mint leaves, washed

Directions

Combine all ingredients in a pitcher and stir. Refrigerate for at least 24 hours. Pour over a glass of ice and enjoy!

---

its metabolism. Instead of using sugar for energy, it uses the other food that you feed it for energy—and best of all it is beginning to burn your fat cells as well.

Train your brain to conquer your cravings

When it comes to eating right, your best ally is within you. No, that's not some new-age drivel. The fact is, you can actually train your brain to deny cravings (or, at least, translate cravings for unhealthy food into healthier choices).

This is a topic I've brought up before, but new research makes it even more compelling… a new study I read examined the question of what happens to your cravings when you don't give in to them.

The authors in this study, called "How Non-Consumption Shapes Desire," concluded that the longer someone goes without something they crave, the weaker the desire for it becomes.

So, "Out of sight, out of mind," clearly isn't just a cliché. But there is a catch…

Simple swaps could put the junk food industry out of business

This "Jedi mind trick" only works if you're able to find a satisfying alternative to the things you're craving.

The researchers found that cravings actually get stronger in people who don't seek out a substitute.

I'm sure the big corporate behemoths that produce America's beloved junk food by the ton are going to put on their heavy-duty earmuffs and ignore this study.

Because if they really took it to heart, they'd realize it could turn their entire industry on its ear. You see, their marketing campaigns directly target cravings…and they build entire campaigns out of creating desire for their products.

Remember the whole Twinkies™ fiasco? Hostess briefly "retired" them (a very happy period, in my book). But just a few months later came the headlines trumpeting their return. "They're finally back! You've been craving them!"

The whole marketing campaign played on the very concepts of "non-consumption and desire." Only they used it in reverse—increasing desire by reminding people that Twinkies were gone.

This is where "training your brain" would have come in handy. If people had found a substitute that satisfied those Twinkie twinges, well, then they wouldn't have felt the need to rush out and re-stock their pantries with them when they made their comeback.

But you don't have to wait for your favorite junk foods to disappear from store shelves to find healthy alternatives for them.

In fact, this can be one of the most fun parts of adopting a healthy new lifestyle.

Practice makes perfect

Think about the things you love to eat…and then figure out ways to make them better for you.

In other words, forget the idea of "deprivation." Thinking about what you "can't" have will only make you miserable and feed those cravings. Instead, focus on shifting your cravings in the right direction.

Visualize all of the wonderfully indulgent foods you CAN enjoy (and still lose weight)—things like juicy burgers dripping with cheese and southern fried chicken with crispy skin. (You can find recipes like these—and many more—in my special report *Dr. Fred's Decadent Diet-Free Recipes*. You can download and view it free by logging in to the Archives on my website, www.drpescatore.com.)

Also, remember: food is just that. *Food*. It's what your body needs to survive. Nothing more. Don't give it any other meaning in your life than that.

Three more tips to keep cravings at bay

I know denying your cravings isn't always easy. It can make you downright cranky. Believe me, I've been there.

So here are a few more things I've found that are great for keeping cravings at bay:

1. Stay hydrated. Drink lots of water throughout your day.

2. Keep moving. Even a little exercise can go a long way in reducing your cravings. I'm not talking about working up a sweat or spending hours in the gym. A walk around the block will do. The idea here is that when you're moving, your brain is otherwise occupied and there's simply no room for those cravings. And you'll be surprised how long the effect lasts.

3. Try glutamine. This amino acid is my go-to rescue remedy for all sorts of things. It provides energy to your muscles and your brain. And it regulates a number of biological functions, including the synthesis of protein, vitamin B3, and the antioxidant glutathione. It's also a world-class craving killer, for a few different reasons.

For starters, it's able to inhibit insulin release, which prevents hard blood-sugar crashes. (The same crashes that often trigger intense cravings.) It also stimulates your body to release stored glucose (called glycogen) in order to get low blood sugar back on track. And finally, glutamine is able to stand in for sugar itself when your body really needs the energy.

In a nutshell, glutamine ensures that your blood sugar never gets low enough that your body hits the panic button. That's why I recommend glutamine to all my dieting patients—500 mg, three times a day, and whenever you get the urge to stick your head into a box of Mallomars.

Don't get me wrong—I think it's important to enjoy your meals. And it's never been easier to do that than with my New Hamptons Health Miracle. But if you're turning to food for comfort, for validation, or for any reason other than sustenance, you'll only wind up hungrier than ever.

So, if you find yourself craving a bag of chips, a cookie, or a pizza, take a deep breath and make a conscious choice not to give in. Try a handful of nuts, some celery dipped in peanut butter, or a few slices of deli meat and some cheese instead. Any one of these will keep you feeling satisfied far longer that what you were originally craving.

And remember, practice makes perfect. Developing new habits isn't easy, but I will be here to help you every step of the way.

Chapter 25

SSC: The SECRET SUPER-CHARGER that makes dodging diabetes simple

There's a top-secret super-food I recommend to all my patients. It's an essential part of my New Hamptons Health Miracle. And can make all the difference between moderate results and a true healing miracle. I've seen it work for thousands of my patients. And it's worked for me as well!

The SSC secret is…Macadamia nut oil.

It's the kicker that changed everything for my patients—multiplying the power of my dietary recommendations. And doing away with the need for steely discipline. Because shedding the weight becomes easier than ever. All they had to do was replace the olive oil they were using with macadamia nut oil.

You can add it to entrees, sides, salads or desserts of every variety, making them even healthier. In my opinion, it blows away olive oil, flaxseed, grape seed or any other oil you may have tried…

Like the genie in "Aladdin's lamp," *it grants three wonderful wishes….*

1. It cleans up blood sludge, helping to lower your total cholesterol and LDL "bad" cholesterol and triglycerides, all while keeping your "good" HDL in check.

2. It promotes healthy blood pressure.

3. And best of all…it helps make you THINNER. Nobody seems to know why yet. But Japanese scientists found when they fed people a macadamia nut-rich diet, it not only helped the patients lose weight, it also reduced their body mass index (BMI). Which means they were losing body fat.

So while olive oil gets all the glory… macadamia nut oil will win hands down, every time. Thanks to its taste, nutrition, and ease and versatility of use.

Macadamia nut oil has the highest amount of monounsaturated fats—with about 80—85 percent. Those fats are one of the secrets of the heart-healthy "Mediterranean" way of eating. Macadamia nut oil is also low in omega-6 fats. These fats are less desirable, because they can cause inflammation. And macadamia nut oil is healthier to cook with thanks to its high smoke point—up to 400 degrees F.

Even a light sauté can reach 350 degrees F, and most unprocessed oils start to break down by that point. Even extra virgin olive oil, whose smoke point is around 320 depending on the kind. In fact, the smoke point of olive oil can vary so much between the types used and the quality, it's difficult to know what you have. This makes even a light sauté with olive oil a gamble.

Macadamia nut oil, on the other hand, is safe for sautéing, baking, even pan frying—however you would want to use oil. There is no danger of those deadly trans-fatty acids and free radicals forming as they can with other cooking oils.

But the real beauty of macadamia nut oil is that it tastes light and buttery. Its flavor isn't overpowering. While it's strong enough to hold its own as a frying oil, it can also easily be used with delicate dishes. Including fish, or as a finishing oil over salads. It's even great in recipes you wouldn't want to ruin with the strong taste of olive oil—things like omelets, muffins, or pancakes.

Macadamia nut oil can still be a little hard to find. Stores like Whole Foods or specialty/gourmet food stores usually have it. You can also find it online.

Easy to use, easy to LOVE!

I learned how to use macadamia nut oil simply by substituting it in my old standard recipes. And wow! What a difference it made! Just start to switch the oil you use in everyday cooking with macadamia nut oil, to create a monounsaturated-rich diet. I promise it will be as if you're eating entirely new delicious foods—that's how much it enhances the flavor of any dish.

You'll love it so much, you'll use it for all your oil needs... I certainly do.

Move Over Mayo!

Want an easy way to get rich (monounsaturated rich, that is)? Swap out your regular mayonnaise with this better-than-the-real-thing version.

Yield: 2 cups

Ingredients
3 egg yolks
juice of 1/2 lemon
1-1/3 cups macadamia nut oil

Directions: Place the yolks and lemon juice in the bowl of a food processor. Turn the machine on, and slowly drizzle in the oil until the mixture is thick and emulsified. Season a portion of the Maconnaise with salt, pepper, and your favorite herb—tarragon, chives, or basil, for example.

Maconnaise Variations

Because Maconnaise is so versatile and because the recipe makes quite a bit of Maconnaise, you can experiment with different flavors by adding to the basic recipe to create many variations and delicious dishes that are rich in monounsaturates. I always keep the basic Maconnaise in my refrigerator and use the following variations when I need a little change. They're all delicious, and you can easily make your own versions.

South of the Border: Mix in 2 seeded and minced chipotle peppers in abobo sauce.

Asian: Mix in 1 1/2 teaspoons freshly grated ginger.

Steak Sauce: Mix in 1 cup finely crumbled blue or gorgonzola cheese.

Dijonnaise: Mix in 1 tablespoon Dijon mustard.

Japanese: Mix in 1 teaspoon wasabi mustard.

Sunday Brunch: Mix in teaspoon horseradish.

Delhi: Mix in 1 teaspoon each cumin and turmeric.

Provencal: Mix in 1 shaving black truffle or 1 teaspoon white truffle oil.

Thai: Mix in a chopped scallion, 2 tablespoons red chili paste, and 1 jalapeno pepper, seeded and chopped.

PART IV

DECADENT DIET-FREE RECIPES

If you've been struggling to eat what you're "supposed" to—only to get fatter and sicker, listen up!

Now, finally, you can forget about depriving yourself. I have made it even easier to indulge your way to a slimmer, healthier, future. You won't believe what's not off limits! Now you can start enjoying your food again, with things like…

- **Deep, Dark & Delicious!** Chocolate deserts
- **15-Minute Weeknight Feasts!**
- **Magnificent Make-aheads!** (And freeze-aheads)
- **Oh Yes, You CAN!** "Diet" impossibilities
- **NO-COOK CUISINE!** Sure to please

And you don't have to banish carbs from your life forever. In fact, certain kinds can actually help you. So get ready to go ahead and banish breakfast boredom forever, long for lunches again, and dine in decadence very night!

To get you started, following are a few general guidelines to keep in mind as you enjoy the recipes to follow.

First…oils you should NEVER cook with!

Even good oils can go bad when they're heated past their smoke point, and each oil has a different smoke point. The following oils should never be heated:

- Flaxseed oil
- Fish oil
- Borage oil
- Evening primrose oil
- Wheat germ oil
- Hemp Seed oil
- Black currant oil

Chapter 26

BREAKFAST:

Never be bored again!

Even Better Than Mom's Oatmeal

4 servings

Ingredients

Pinch of Salt

2-1/2 cups water

1 cup steel-cut oats

1/3 cup lo-han, or Stevia to taste *(optional)*

1/2 teaspoon cinnamon, ground

2 tablespoons Tabasco sauce

1/2 cup cheddar cheese, shredded

Directions

In a large saucepan bring the salted water to a rolling boil. Add oats and cook for about 20 minutes, stirring constantly. Transfer the oats from the saucepan to a large mixing bowl and add the remaining ingredients except the cheese. Mix thoroughly. Divide the mixture into four bowls and sprinkle equally with the grated cheese. You could serve the oatmeal immediately this way, or you could place the (heatproof) bowls under the broiler until the cheese gets crispy.

Craveable Crab Quiche

6 servings

Ingredients

2 tablespoons macadamia nut oil + macadamia nut oil spray

4 green onions, chopped into a fine dice

12 ounces fresh crabmeat

1 teaspoon grated lemon rind, rated

1/2 teaspoon Old Bay Seasoning

1/8 teaspoon ground red pepper

1 cup heavy whipping cream

3 large eggs

1/2 teaspoon black pepper

1/2 teaspoon salt

6 ounces parmesan cheese, grated

Directions

Preheat oven to 400 degrees. Heat oil in a large skillet and saute the first five ingredients together for 2–3 minutes. Whisk together the cream, eggs, and spices in a large bowl. Stir in crabmeat mixture and cheese. Pour into a nonstick 9-inch pie pan that has been sprayed with macadamia nut oil. Place on the lowest rack of the oven and bake for 40 minutes or until set. Let stand for 10 minutes before removing from the pan and placing on a serving dish.

Creamy-Dreamy Pine Nut Muffins

6 servings

Ingredients

1 cup ricotta cheese

2 large eggs

1/2 cup parmesan cheese, grated

1/2 teaspoon salt

2 packets Stevia

1/2 teaspoon vanilla extract

1 ounce pignoli nuts, toasted and crushed

Directions

Preheat oven to 350 degrees. In a medium bowl, combine the ricotta and eggs and mix until smooth. Add the parmesan, salt, Stevia, and vanilla. Mix again until smooth. Mix the nuts throughout the batter. Pour into a nonstick muffin pan and bake for 15 to 20 minutes.

Mouth-watering Macadamia Pancakes— Blueberry, too!

4 servings

Ingredients

1/2 cup almond flour or soy protein isolate

3 eggs

1/4 cup water

1/4 cup heavy cream

2 ounces crushed macadamia nuts (or 2 ounces blueberries)

1/4 teaspoon salt

Macadamia nut oil

Directions

Combine the first six ingredients in a mixing bowl and mix thoroughly with a whisk. Note that there should be lumps. Spray a large skillet or griddle with a light coating of oil. When the oil is hot, pour about 1 tablespoon of the batter onto the griddle or skillet, cooking evenly on both sides, about 1 minute for each. Continue until all the batter is used.

Crispy Corned Beef Hash

4 servings

Ingredients

1 (3-pound) corned beef

1 cup cabbage, shredded

1 dill pickle

Salt

Pepper

2 tablespoons macadamia nut oil

4 ounces cheddar cheese, grated

Directions

Place the corned beef in a large stock pot, and cover with water. Bring to a boil, reduce the heat to simmer, cover, and cook for 3 hours. Add the shredded cabbage to the water, and simmer for another 30 minutes. Remove the beef from the pot, and allow to rest until it can be handled. Remove any excess fat or gristle. Drain the cabbage, and set aside. Puree the dill pickle in a blender or a food processor. Cube half the corned beef and shred the other half. In a large bowl, mix the corned beef, pickle, and cabbage. Season to taste. In a large skillet, heat the oil until warm over medium-high heat. Add the corned beef mixture, and press down with a spatula. Cook until crisp, turning once. Divide the hash among four plates, sprinkle the cheese over each dish, and serve.

Scrumptious Sausage Scramble

4 servings

Ingredients

1-1/2 cups heavy cream

4 tablespoons parmesan cheese, freshly grated

Macadamia nut oil spray

1/4 pound hot pork sausage, crumbled

1 tablespoon macadamia nut oil

1 green onion, very thinly sliced

1 green pepper, roasted and peeled, cut into thin strips

1 jalapeno, seeded and finely minced

1 clove garlic, finely minced

Kosher salt

10 eggs

8 ounces shredded Monterey Jack cheese

Freshly ground black pepper

Directions

Combine cream and parmesan in a medium bowl, and whisk until frothy. In a large skillet, spray a little oil and add the sausage, cooking over high heat until browned, about 4 minutes. Set on paper towels, and drain excess fat from skillet. Add the tablespoon of oil and heat. When hot, add the onion, roasted green pepper, jalapeno, garlic, and salt. Cook over medium-high heat until the onions are translucent, about 5 minutes. Remove from heat, and add the sausage, eggs, 1 1/3 cup cheese, and black pepper, and mix well. Spray a 10-inch baking dish with the oil to lightly cover. Sprinkle 1/3 cup cheese onto the bottom of the baking dish. Pour in the egg mixture, being careful to distribute the ingredients evenly. Sprinkle the remaining cheese on top, and bake in a preheated 350-degree F oven for about 60 minutes or until a toothpick inserted in the center comes out clean.

Scrumptious Sausage Scramble (continued)

To Grill a Pepper — Cut into strips, remove the seeds, arrange on a foil-lined baking sheet, and broil until blackened, about 8 minutes. Remove from heat, wrap the foil around the pepper and allow to steam. When cool enough to handle, remove the skins. This method can be used to roast any type of pepper. The timing may be a little more or a little less, depending on the variety.

Spicy Huevos Benedict

8 servings

Ingredients

Chipotle hollandaise Sauce (see next recipe)

8 large eggs, poached

2 cup shredded Monterey Jack cheese with peppers

1 cup salsa—your favorite salsa will do here, as long as it doesn't contain sugar

8 teaspoons sour cream

Directions

Ladle a small portion of the hollandaise sauce onto each plate. Then put the poached egg onto the center of the plate, place some shredded cheeses and salsa on top of each egg, drizzle more of the hollandaise sauce on each egg, and top with a dollop of sour cream.

OH YES YOU CAN!

Chipotle Hollandaise Sauce

Yields 1-1/2 cups

Ingredients

4 large egg yolks

2 tablespoons fresh lemon juice

1 cup butter, melted

1 tablespoon fresh minced cilantro

4 teaspoons pureed chipotle peppers in adobo sauce.
This ingredient can be found in the international section of
your supermarket or in Latin grocery stores in a can.

1/4 teaspoon salt

Directions

Whisk the yolks in the top of a double boiler, then gradually whisk in
the lemon juice. Place over hot water that's in the bottom of the double
boiler (do not boil). Add butter, 1/3 cup at a time, whisk in until smooth;
whisk in the cilantro; whisk until smooth; whisk in the peppers and then
the salt. Cook, whisking constantly, about 10 minutes or until thickened
and a thermometer registers 160 degrees F. Serve immediately.

Berry-Kissed Breakfast Shake

1 serving

Ingredients

> 2 ripe strawberries, cut into small pieces
>
> 2 ounces heavy whipping cream
>
> 8 ounces water
>
> 1 scoop almond or whey protein powder (unsweetened)
>
> Ice
>
> 1 tablespoon macadamia nut oil

Directions

Combine all ingredients in a blender and liquefy. I add the macadamia nut oil to this recipe because a tablespoon a day may keep the doctor away. You can choose not to add this, but it makes the drink extra rich and smooth.

Bubbling-Over Spinach Pie

6 servings

Ingredients

1 pound Italian sausage

1 (10-ounce) package frozen chopped spinach, thawed

1 (15-ounce) container ricotta cheese

1 (8-ounce) package cream cheese

4 ounces shredded mozzarella

2 eggs, beaten

1/2 teaspoon hot sauce

2 teaspoons Italian seasonings

Directions

Preheat oven to 400 degrees F. Cook and crumble the sausage. Drain the spinach and squeeze it dry. Combine all ingredients. Butter a 10-inch pie plate and smooth mixture in plate. Bake for 40 minutes until set and light golden brown. Cool for 5 minutes before cutting into wedges.

Buttery Bistro Avocado & Brie Omelet

4 servings

Ingredients

6 eggs

1-1/2 ounces grated Parmesan cheese

Salt

1 tablespoon unsalted butter

Filling

1/4 cup minced ham

1 ounce Brie, cubed without the rind

2 ounces avocado, sliced

Directions

Preheat oven to 375 degrees F. Beat the eggs with a pinch of salt and the cheese. Grease a jelly roll pan with butter, cover the butter with parchment paper and butter the parchment paper (as an easy alternative, you can spray the parchment with macadamia nut oil). Pour the egg mixture over the parchment and bake for 10 minutes. Remove the egg roll-up from the pan and spread with the ingredients for the filling. Roll the egg sheet as you would a jelly roll. Slice and serve.

Savory Sicilian Egg Roll-up

4 servings

Ingredients

6 eggs

1-1/2 ounces grated Parmesan cheese

Salt

1 tablespoon unsalted butter

Filling

1/4 cup cooked Italian sausage, crumbled

1/2 ounce shredded provolone cheese

1 teaspoon oregano

1 tablespoon minced tomatoes

Directions

Preheat oven to 375 degrees F. Beat the eggs with a pinch of salt and the cheese. Grease a jelly roll pan with butter, cover the butter with parchment paper and butter the parchment paper (as an easy alternative, you can spray the parchment with macadamia nut oil). Pour the egg mixture over the parchment and bake for 10 minutes. Remove the egg roll-up from the pan and spread with the ingredients for the filling. Roll the egg sheet as you would a jelly roll. Slice and serve.

Chapter 27

LUNCH:

Enjoy all these "forbidden" favorites!

Southwestern BLT

1 serving

Ingredients

4 slices turkey bacon (thin)

2 slices whole grain bread

1 tablespoon maconnaise (see recipe on the next page)

1 chipotle chili, minced

1/4 cup avocado (mashed or sliced)

2 slices tomato

2 leaves of lettuce

Directions

Fry the turkey bacon until it's crisp and drain. Toast the whole grain bread. Wisk together the maconnaise and chipotle chili in a bowl. Spread the chipotle maconnaise and avocado on both slices of the whole grain toast. Then build your sandwich with the tomatoes, lettuce and bacon. Slice down the center and serve.

Maconnaise

Want an easy way to get rich (monounsaturated rich, that is)? Swap out your regular mayonnaise with this better-than-the-real-thing version.

Yield: 2 cups

Ingredients

3 egg yolks
juice of 1/2 lemon
1-1/3 cups macadamia nut oil

Directions

Place the yolks and lemon juice in the bowl of a food processor. Turn the machine on, and slowly drizzle in the oil until the mixture is thick and emulsified. Season a portion of the Maconnaise with salt, pepper, and your favorite herb—tarragon, chives, or basil, for example.

Magnificent Make-Ahead!

Artichoke and Shrimp Chowder

8 servings

Ingredients

3 tablespoons macadamia nut oil

1 small onion, finely chopped

2 garlic cloves, minced

3 ribs celery, peeled and cut along the diagonal into a small dice

1 (6-ounce) can artichoke hearts

24 ounces reduced-sodium chicken broth, organic

1 teaspoon dried thyme

1 bay leaf

1 teaspoon red pepper

4 ounces heavy cream

kosher salt

pepper

2 tablespoons cauliflower puree

1 pound small uncooked shrimp

1/2 cup chopped cilantro for garnish

Directions

In a large stockpot, heat the oil and all the onion, garlic, celery, and artichoke hearts, then sauté for about 5 minutes until the onion is translucent. Gradually stir in the broth, and bring to a simmer. Add all the other ingredients except the shrimp and cilantro leaves, and simmer for one hour, allowing it to reduce. Add 1 tablespoon of cauliflower puree or continue to simmer for another 30 minutes. Finally, add the shrimp, cook for 10 minutes, and serve garnished with cilantro leaves.

Savory Stuffed Peppers

6 servings

Ingredients

6 medium-sized Italian green frying peppers

1 pound ground chuck

1 medium onion

2 cloves garlic

1 cup shredded parmesan cheese

1/4 teaspoon crushed red pepper

1/2 teaspoon salt

1/2 teaspoon pepper

macadamia nut oil, as needed

Directions

Cut the top off the peppers, and remove the innards, including the seeds. Cook ground beef in a large skillet over medium heat, about 6 minutes, stirring until the beef crumbles. Add the onion and garlic, and sauté 4 or more minutes or until the beef is no longer pink. Remove from heat and drain. Stir in the crushed red pepper, salt and black pepper. Spoon the mixture evenly into the frying peppers, and place in a baking dish that has been lightly coated with oil. Sprinkle the parmesan cheese over the peppers, lightly drizzle some macadamia nut oil on top, and place on a pre-heated 350 degree F oven for about 20 minutes to make sure the peppers get soft but do not burn on the top. Cover with foil, if needed, at this time.

Sinfully Smothered Hot Dogs

8 servings

Ingredients

8 hot dogs, preferably organic and without preservatives

4 ounces cheddar cheese, shredded

1/2 cup salsa

1 cup iceberg lettuce, shredded

Sour cream (if desired)

Guacamole (if desired)

Directions

Cook hot dogs in boiling water for 5 minutes. Combine the cheese and salsa in a glass bowl, and microwave on high for 1 minute or until thoroughly heated, stirring once. Cut a small slit on one side of the hot dog so that it lies flat on the plate. Spread the heated mixture on top of the hot dogs, and top evenly with shredded lettuce, sour cream, and guacamole.

The Happy Snack

Macadamia nuts aren't just delicious and good for your body, they're also good for your mood. Macadamia nuts are a rich source of tyrosine, a precursor of serotonin, the "happy" brain chemical.

Luscious Lemon-Tarragon Chicken Salad

2 servings

Ingredients

2 cups chicken broth

1 pound boneless, skinless chicken breast

1/2 cup Maconnaise (see recipe on page 267)

2 tablespoons Dijon mustard

2 radicchio leaves

4 teaspoons lemon juice

2 teaspoons lemon peel

2 tablespoons minced fresh tarragon, or 2 teaspoons dried

1/2 cup diced celery

Directions

Bring the chicken broth to a simmer in a large saucepan. Add the chicken breasts and simmer until cooked through and no longer pink, about 7 to 10 minutes. Remove from the broth and cool. Once cool, shred the chicken. Reserve 1/2 cup of the broth and discard the rest. In a small, nonreactive bowl, combine the next five ingredients to make the dressing. To thin the dressing, add chicken broth two tablespoons at a time until the desired consistency is reached. Mix together the shredded chicken, celery, and dressing. Mound on radicchio leaf to serve.

Heavenly Ham Casserole

6 servings

Ingredients

1 medium cauliflower

4 tablespoons butter

1 cup heavy whipping cream

4 ounces cheddar cheese, shredded

1/2 cup sour cream

2 cups cubed cooked ham

1 cup mushrooms, sliced

1 cup parmesan cheese, grated

1 tablespoon cold butter

Directions

Preheat oven to 350 degrees. Cut cauliflower into florets and cook in boiling salted water for about 10 minutes or until tender; drain and set aside. Melt the 4 tablespoons of butter in a medium saucepan over medium heat. Do not let it burn. Slowly add the heavy cream, whisking constantly until the mixture starts to reduce and thicken slightly. Add the cheddar cheese and sour cream, stirring until the cheese melts, but do not let it boil. Stir in the cauliflower, ham, and mushrooms and pour into a 2-quart baking dish. Sprinkle the parmesan cheese evenly over the casserole. Cut 1 tablespoon of cold butter into pieces, and sprinkle over the parmesan. Bake uncovered for 45 minutes.

Impossibly Creamy Squash Soup

8 servings

Ingredients

1/4 cup macadamia nut oil

8 cups yellow squash, diced

4 stalks celery, with leaves, diced

1 medium onion, diced

64 ounces organic chicken broth or homemade
   organic chicken stock

1 pint heavy cream

1/2 cup Parmesan cheese

Black pepper, freshly ground Salt, to taste

Directions

Over medium heat, add the macadamia nut oil to a large soup pot. Add the squash, celery, and onion. Cover and cook until the vegetables are soft and the squash starts to break down. Add the chicken broth and simmer until the broth reduces by half. Add the heavy cream and Parmesan cheese and mix thoroughly. Just before serving, add pepper, and taste the soup to see if it needs any salt. This may be served with a small dollop of sour cream or a pinch of cayenne pepper.

Seafarer's Secret Shrimp Salad

6 servings

Ingredients

2 tablespoons macadamia nut oil

1/2 red bell pepper, seeded, de-ribbed, and diced

1/2 cup chopped fresh parsley

2 tablespoons Dijon mustard

1/4 cup Maconnaise (see recipe on page 267)

1/2 cup sour cream

1 tablespoon fresh lime juice

1 teaspoon fresh tarragon, minced

1 pound small shrimp, boiled (can buy already cooked fresh or frozen, thawed)

Sea salt

Freshly ground white pepper

5 heads Belgian endive

Directions

Mix the pepper, parsley, mustard, Maconnaise, sour cream, lime juice, and tarragon until well combined. Add the shrimp, and mix gently. Season with salt and pepper to taste. Separate the leaves of the endive, and select 36 of the best leaves. Put 1 tablespoon of the mixture onto each leaf, and arrange on a plate. Each plate gets 6 filled leaves. Sprinkle each plate with additional tarragon, and serve.

Rich & Robust Roast Beef Wraps

6 servings

Ingredients

> 1 medium red onion, halved and sliced
>
> 1 yellow bell pepper, halved and sliced
>
> 6 romaine lettuce leaves
>
> Mustard-Horseradish Crème (see next recipe)
>
> 1 pound roast beef, thinly sliced

Directions

> Lay out the large lettuce leaves, one per plate. Spread the Mustard-Horseradish Crème onto each leaf. Next, lay the roast beef into each leaf. Divide the bell pepper and onion mixture evenly into each leaf and onto the roast beef, then finish with the remaining mustard mixture. (This is also good if you sauté the onions and pepper in a little macadamia nut oil first!)

Mustard-Horseradish Crème

Yields 1 cup

Ingredients

> 1 cup sour cream or crème fraiche
>
> 3 tablespoons horseradish
>
> 1 teaspoon dry mustard
>
> 1/4 teaspoon lemon rind

Directions

> Stir together all ingredients in a small bowl. Chill until ready to serve.

Gift of the Gods Greek Lettuce Boats

6 servings

Ingredients

1/2 pound fresh mozzarella, cut into 1/2-inch pieces

1 cup macadamia nut oil and red wine vinegar dressing

1/2 cup kalamata olives, pitted and halved

2 green onions, sliced

2 tablespoons chopped fresh basil

1 tablespoon chopped fresh thyme

1/4 teaspoon pepper

6 large outer romaine lettuce leaves

1 pound thinly sliced fresh turkey breast

10 bacon slices, cooked and crumbled

3 cups chopped romaine lettuce

Directions

Combine the mozzarella and the dressing in a shallow dish or a resealable plastic bag; cover or seal, and chill for 1 hour. Toss together the olives, the next four ingredients, and the mozzarella mixture. Let stand for 20 minutes. Lay out the large lettuce leaves on each plate, and divide the turkey evenly among the leaves. Then divide the mixture among the turkey/lettuce boats, and sprinkle each one with bacon and the chopped romaine leaves.

Maine Lobster Rolls

Serves 4

Ingredients

- 1 tablespoon butter, softened
- 4 whole grain hot dog buns or Kaiser rolls, split (if you can't find whole grain rolls, you can also use tortilla wraps or whole grain baguette)
- 4 lettuce leaves
- 1-1/2 pounds cooked and cubed lobster meat
- 2 tablespoons maconnaise (see recipe page 267)
- 1 teaspoon fresh lime juice
- 1 dash Tabasco™
- 2 green onions, chopped
- 1 stalk celery, finely chopped
- Salt and pepper to taste
- 1 pinch dried basil, parsley or tarragon

Directions

Lightly butter the insides of the buns or rolls and line with lettuce leaves. Set aside. In a medium bowl, stir together the maconnaise, lime juice, hot pepper sauce, salt and pepper until well blended. Mix in the green onion and celery, then lightly mix in the lobster so it just gets coated without falling apart. Stuff the lobster filling into the buns and sprinkle parsley, basil or tarragon lightly over the filling.

Chapter 28

DINNERS:
Dine in decadence!

Fall-Off-Your-Fork Pork Tenderloin

8 servings

Ingredients

4 tablespoons macadamia nut oil

3/4 pound of your favorite mushrooms, sliced

1 small onion, chopped

1/4 cup chopped pecans, toasted

2 (12-ounce) pork tenderloins, flattened to 1/4-inch thickness

1 teaspoon salt

1 teaspoon fresh ground black pepper

8 thick bacon slices

Macadamia nut oil spray

1 teaspoon fresh cracked black pepper

Directions

Heat the oil in a large skillet over medium-high heat, add the mushrooms and onion, and sauté for 8 to 10 minutes or until tender. Stir in the pecans, and set aside. Flatten the pork loins or have the butcher do this for you, to 1/4-inch thickness. To do this yourself, you'll need a rolling pin or a meat mallet. After flattening, sprinkle with salt and ground pepper. Spread the mushroom mixture evenly on one side of the tenderloin, leaving a 1/4-inch border. Roll it up jellyroll-style, starting with the long end, and wrap 4 bacon slices around each tenderloin. Secure with toothpicks, and place on a lightly oil-sprayed rack in a roasting pan, seam sides down. Rub with the cracked pepper. Bake uncovered in a preheated 450-degree F oven for 15 minutes. Reduce the temperature to 400 degrees F, and cook for another 15 minutes.

Magnificent Make-Ahead!

Divine Chicken Devon

4 servings

Ingredients

3 tablespoons macadamia nut oil

4 boneless, skinless chicken breast halves, flattened

Kosher salt

Fresh ground white pepper

1 shallot, chopped

1 tablespoon fresh chopped tarragon

1/2 cup heavy whipping cream

Fresh-squeezed lemon juice, to taste

Chopped fresh Italian parsley for garnish

Directions

Heat the oil in a large skillet over medium-high heat. Season the chicken with salt and pepper. When the oil is heated, add the chicken and sauté gently on each side, turning once, until the juices run clear, about 3 minutes per side. Transfer to a heated plate, and place in a food warmer. Pour off any excess fat from the skillet, and return to medium heat. Add the shallot, and sauté for about 1-1/2 minutes. Add the tarragon and the cream, increase the heat, and stir, getting the browned bits on the bottom of the pan. Blend well. Continue stirring until mixture is bubbling, about 3 minutes. Do not burn. Sauce should be starting to thicken by this time. Season with salt, pepper, and a squeeze of lemon juice. Return the chicken to the pan, and coat well on each side. Put on individual plates, and lightly drizzle sauce over each breast. Sprinkle with the fresh parsley and serve.

"Cheater's" Chicken Cutlets

4 servings

Ingredients

1 teaspoon cayenne pepper

2 cups freshly grated parmesan

2 eggs

1/2 cup heavy cream

Kosher salt

Freshly ground black pepper

Macadamia oil for frying

2 pounds boneless, skinless chicken breasts, pounded thin

Directions

Combine the cayenne and parmesan on a plate. Beat eggs in a bowl with the heavy cream, salt, and pepper. In a large skillet, pour oil to a depth of about 1/4 inch. Dip the breasts into the parmesan, then into the egg, and then back into the parmesan. Place on another plate until each breast has been coated. Heat the oil on medium-high heat, and do not put the chicken in until the oil is very hot. You'll know when it's ready if you drop a small piece of the parmesan coating into the oil and it begins to sizzle. This is the key to making the chicken cutlets without breading. Place the chicken cutlets in the oil and allow to cook thoroughly on the first side before turning. They are not ready to turn until the side facing you starts to look as if it's cooking. Use a spatula to carefully turn the chicken and allow to cook until the top side is golden brown. Remove to a plate and serve.

Grill-Lover's Rib-eye Steak Salad

8 servings

Ingredients

4 (8-ounce) rib-eye steaks

Salt to taste

Pepper to taste

1 teaspoon fresh chopped thyme

1 teaspoon fresh chopped basil

2 teaspoons ground cumin

Macadamia nut oil spray

3 romaine lettuce hearts

Salad Dressing (recipe follows)

1 medium red onion, slice into very thin rings

Directions

Season the steaks with salt and pepper. Place the thyme, basil, and cumin in a small dish. Spray the steaks with a light coating of macadamia nut oil, and rub them in the spice mixture. Allow to season for at least 2 hours or up to 24 hours, if preferred.

Preheat the grill. Grill the steaks to desired doneness, about 8 minutes on each side for medium, and keep them warm. Divide the romaine leaves onto eight plates. Dress the salads individually, then slice the steaks thinly and arrange on the salad. Before serving, put two slices of red onion on top of each steak, add another dollop of dressing, and serve.

Scrumptious Beef Stroganoff

6 servings

Ingredients

2 pounds filet of beef

Salt and pepper

4 tablespoons butter

1 tablespoon almond flour

2 cups beef broth

2 tablespoons tomato paste

2 tablespoons sour cream

1/4 cup grated onion

2 tablespoons minced parsley

Directions

Cut the beef into thin strips and generously sprinkle with salt and pepper. Allow the beef to rest in the refrigerator for one hour.

Melt 2 tablespoons of the butter in a small saucepan. Add the almond flour and stir until smooth. Slowly add the beef broth and stir with a whisk to prevent lumps. Boil for 2 minutes. Stirring constantly, add the tomato paste and sour cream. Simmer gently.

In a nonstick frying pan, sauté the onion in the remaining butter until translucent. Add the strips of beef and fry until brown. Add the broth mixture and cover the pan. Simmer gently for 30 minutes. Garnish with the parsley.

Southern Fried Chicken with Crispy Skin

4 servings

Ingredients

3 to 6 cups macadamia nut oil (depending on pot used)

1 whole chicken, cut into 8 pieces,
   or 3 pounds boneless chicken breast

3 eggs

1/4 cup heavy cream or water

Breading

2 1/3 cups oat or almond flour

2 teaspoons salt

1 teaspoon black pepper

1 teaspoon garlic powder

1 teaspoon poultry seasoning

Directions

Preheat oven to 350 degrees F. Place a heavy pot over medium-high heat with at least 1-inch of macadamia nut oil for boneless chicken and 2 inches for whole pieces. Heat oil to 350 degrees F; it is important to monitor and maintain the temperature, or the almond flour breading and your oil will burn. In a medium bowl, mix the eggs and cream to make an egg wash. In a separate larger bowl, mix all the breading ingredients together. Season the chicken well with salt and pepper. Dip it first in the breading, then in the egg wash, and then back in the breading again, making sure to coat well on all sides. Pat off any excess breading and then carefully place into hot oil and fry until golden brown and crisp, just a few minutes. Remove and drain on paper towels. Boneless chicken breasts, if thinly cut, may cook all the way by frying alone, but whole chicken will not because of how fast almond flour browns. It is best to place any chicken you fry with almond flour on a sheet pan and finish by baking at 350 degrees F for an additional 10 minutes for boneless chicken and 20 to 25 minutes more for cut up chicken pieces that have bones. The internal temperature of the chicken should register 165 degrees F.

Sticky-Finger Spare Ribs

6 servings

Ingredients

2 pounds spare ribs (beef or pork)

2 tablespoons sugar-free soy sauce

1 teaspoon cayenne, chili powder, or a combination of the two

1 tablespoon dried thyme

2 tablespoons dried rosemary

15 drops liquid Stevia

1 teaspoon salt

1 clove garlic, grated

3 tablespoons olive oil

Directions

Put ribs in a roasting pan. Combine all the other ingredients in a bowl and mix thoroughly. Pour over the ribs, and rub them so all sides are coated in the mixture. Place in a 375 degree oven, basting the ribs every 15 minutes. If the sauce runs dry, add some water to the bottom of the pan and continue to baste. Bake for about 1 hour, or until crispy on the outside.

Dr. Fred's Foolproof Secret BBQ Sauce

Ingredients

1 cup yellow mustard

1/2 cup Stevia

3/4 cup cider vinegar

2 tablespoons chili powder

1 teaspoon ground black pepper

1 teaspoon ground white pepper

1/4 teaspoon cayenne pepper

1/2 teaspoon soy sauce

2 tablespoons butter

1 tablespoon liquid smoke flavoring

Directions

In a saucepan over medium heat, stir together the mustard, Stevia, cider vinegar, chili powder, black pepper, white pepper, and cayenne pepper. Simmer for 30 minutes. Stir in the soy sauce, butter, and liquid smoke; simmer for another 10 minutes. Allow the sauce to cool completely, and then refrigerate it overnight to allow the flavors to blend before using.

Succulent Scallops with Crispy Pancetta

4 servings

Ingredients

16 large sea scallops

3 tablespoons macadamia nut oil

6 thin slices pancetta

1 handful baby arugula

1 s
mall head butter lettuce,
torn into larger pieces

1 teaspoon lemon zest

2 tablespoons chopped fennel fronds

2 teaspoons red wine vinegar

Salt

Directions

Preheat your grill to medium. Brush the scallops lightly with the oil. Cut the pancetta to fit around the scallops' rims. Wrap a strip of pancetta around each scallop. In a large stainless steel bowl, toss together the arugula, butter lettuce, lemon zest, and fennel. Sprinkle with the vinegar, and salt to taste. Mix thoroughly, and adjust seasonings as desired. Divide the salad among the four plates. Season the scallops with slat on both sides, and grill until the pancetta is crisp on the edges and the scallops are cooked through, about 5 to 8 minutes. Remove from the grill, and place on top of the salads.

Dripping-with-Cheese Mushroom Burger

4 servings

Ingredients

1 pound ground chuck (85% lean)—anything leaner will
cause drier burgers

Kosher salt

Freshly ground black pepper

3 tablespoons minced scallion,
white part only

1 tablespoon grated fresh ginger

1 cup crumbled blue cheese

2 tablespoons macadamia nut oil

1/2 cup chopped onion

1 garlic clove, minced

3/4 pound chopped white mushrooms

Spinach leaves (raw)

Directions

In a stainless steel bowl, combine the first five ingredients (up to the
cheese), until mixed well. Form this mixture into 8 hamburger patties.
Press an equal amount of cheese on 4 of the patties, and refrigerate. In
the meantime, heat the oil in a small skillet, add the onion and garlic,
and sauté for 5 minutes. Then add the mushrooms, and cook for about
7 minutes or until the mushrooms release their juices. Drain, remove the
burgers from the refrigerator, evenly divide the mushroom/onion/garlic
mixture among the four burgers, then cover with the other 4 patties.
Seal the edges with your fingers, and refrigerate again. On a preheated
medium-high grill, sear each side for 3 to 4 minutes for medium or until
they reach desired doneness. Serve on a bed of spinach leaves.

Herb-and-Cabernet Pot Roast

4 servings

Ingredients

1 cup Cabernet Sauvignon wine

1.5 pounds raw top sirloin roast

2 cloves garlic, minced

Pinch of salt

Pepper, freshly ground

1 teaspoon dried marjoram

1 teaspoon thyme

1 teaspoon oregano leaves

2 sprigs fresh rosemary

1 red onion, quartered and sliced

1-1/2 cups fresh green beans

Directions

Put the roast in a large Ziploc bag or small dish, submerge in the wine, seal and refrigerate overnight. In the morning, put the marinated roast and wine in the bottom of the slow cooker—it's important that the meat is on the bottom, in the liquid, so that it doesn't dry out in the cooking process. Add the garlic, a pinch of salt, a generous amount of freshly ground black pepper, dried marjoram, thyme, oregano and rosemary. Cover with the onion and green beans. Cover the pot, turn on low and let cook for 8-10 hours. Remove the rosemary before serving.

Tempting Taco Salad

6 servings

Ingredients

4 tablespoons macadamia nut oil

1 pound ground beef

1 small onion, chopped

1 garlic clove, minced

1 tablespoon fajita seasoning mix

1 12-ounce jar salsa verde

1/2 head iceberg lettuce, shredded

Guacamole

Sour cream (if desired)

Directions

In a large skillet, heat half the oil over medium-high heat. Add the beef, stirring until the beef crumbles and is no longer pink, about 8 minutes. Drain, pat dry with paper towels, and set aside. In the same skillet, heat the remaining half of the oil, add the onion and the garlic, and sauté for 1 minute. Return the beef to the skillet; add the fajita seasonings and half the salsa verde. Cook over medium-high heat 3 minutes or until thoroughly heated and the liquid has evaporated. Divide the shredded lettuce among 6 plates, pour the beef mixture onto the lettuce; top with guacamole, the remaining salsa verde, and a dollop of sour cream, if desired.

Beef and Goat Cheese Ravioli

4 Servings

Ingredients

1 pound ground beef

1 package wonton skins

1-1/2 cups spinach (fresh)

5 tablespoons fresh grated parmesan cheese

1 cup soft goat cheese

1-1/4 tablespoons parsley (dried)

1/4 cup bread crumbs

1/4 cup macadamia nut oil

1 large egg

1/2 teaspoon garlic salt

1 pinch black pepper

Directions

Heat a large skillet over medium-high heat and stir in the ground beef. Cook and stir until the beef is crumbly, evenly browned, and no longer pink. Drain and discard any excess grease. Stir in the spinach and cook until wilted, about 1 to 2 minutes. Remove from heat and allow to cool for 10 minutes. Transfer the beef mixture to a bowl. Add the Parmesan, parsley, macadamia nut oil, egg, garlic salt, goat cheese and pepper and mix well. Run the filling through a grinder until smooth (or puree in a food processor until smooth). The filling can be kept in the refrigerator for up to four days or in the freezer for up to three months. Lay out wonton skins and brush all sides with macadamia nut oil. Spoon a small mound of filling in the middle of the wonton and place second skin on top. Press firmly together. In 2 quarts of salted, boiling water, blanch raviolis.

Butter-Drenched Lobster

6 servings

Ingredients

6 one-pound lobsters
2 sticks salted butter
Juice of 1 lemon

Directions

Plunge lobsters headfirst into a large pot of boiling water. Cook 12 minutes or until shells are bright red and tails are curled. Remove from water. Meanwhile, melt butter in a saucepan over medium heat. Add lemon juice and stir. Serve lobsters with lemon butter for dipping.

Wedding Banquet Prime Rib

6 servings

Ingredients

1 three-rib prime-rib roast
2 tablespoons macadamia nut oil
2 tablespoons coarse salt
1 tablespoon garlic powder

Directions

Preheat oven to 450 degrees. Rub roast with oil, salt, and garlic powder. Place in a heavy metal roasting pan, fat side up. Cook 20 minutes and then reduce heat to 325. Continue cooking for another hour to hour and a half, or until an instant-read thermometer registers 145 degrees. Transfer the roast to a large platter and set aside. Pour off the juices before slicing and serving.

Island Getaway
Macadamia & Coconut-Crusted Salmon

4 servings

Ingredients

4-5 tablespoons macadamia nut oil

1/4 cup macadamia nuts, crushed, unsalted

1/4 cup coconut flakes, unsweetened

1 tablespoon garlic, minced

1 teaspoon sea salt

1 teaspoon black pepper, freshly ground

4 salmon fillets (wild Alaskan, if possible), skin removed

4 slices lemon

Directions

Preheat the oven to 350 degrees F. On the stove, heat 2 tablespoons of macadamia nut oil to a medium temperature in an ovenproof pan. In a bowl, combine the macadamia nuts, coconut, garlic, salt, and pepper. Rub 1 tablespoon of oil onto the salmon fillets, then press the dry ingredients onto both sides of the salmon. Sauté one side of the salmon fillets in oil. Flip them over in the pan and then put the pan in the oven. For rare, 3 to 4 minutes is all it takes. For more well-done fillets, leave in the oven for 10 minutes. Garnish with lemon and more oil as needed. (You may also top with Hollandaise Sauce, see recipe on page 261, just leave out the chipotle.)

Spicy, Creamy & Saucy Buffalo Meatballs

2 servings

Ingredients

1 pound ground organic buffalo

1 egg

1/4 cup grated Parmesan cheese

1/2 teaspoon salt

1/4 cup chopped Italian parsley

2 tablespoons chopped roasted red pepper

1 jalapeno pepper, seeded and diced

Macadamia nut oil

1 cup button mushrooms, sliced

1/2 pint organic heavy cream

Salt

Black pepper, freshly ground

3 big handfuls of baby spinach

Directions

In a large bowl, mix together the buffalo, egg, cheese, salt, parsley, and red and jalapeno peppers. You may adjust the amount of jalapeno depending on your individual taste. Form meatballs about the size of golf balls. Place them in a cast-iron skillet with some macadamia nut oil. Sauté and turn as needed until the meatballs are cooked through. While the meatballs are cooking, sauté the mushrooms in a saucepan with some macadamia nut oil until they are cooked down. Place the mushrooms into a blender with the cream and blend until a sauce forms. Salt and pepper the sauce to taste. On a serving plate, form a bed out of the baby spinach. Top the spinach with the meatballs. Pour the cream sauce over the meatballs and serve. The heat from the buffalo meatballs and mushroom sauce will wilt the spinach.

Rib-Sticking Korean Short Ribs

2 servings

Ingredients

1-1/2 pounds flanken-style beef short ribs, 1/2 inch thick

Marinade

1 teaspoon sesame seeds

1/4 cup tamari sauce

1/4 cup water

2 teaspoons sesame oil

2 teaspoons minced fresh ginger

2 cloves garlic, minced

1 teaspoon garlic powder

1/2 teaspoon freshly ground black pepper

1/2 cup minced scallions

Directions

Put all of the marinade ingredients into a blender and whirl to combine. Put the ribs into a self-closing plastic bag, pour the marinade over the ribs, and close the bag. Refrigerate at least overnight and up to 2 days. The longer the ribs are allowed to marinate, the more flavorful they will be. Heat the grill. Drain the ribs and discard the marinade. Grill about 1-1/2 minutes per side. Serve hot.

Fantastically Fresh Tomato Bread salad with Country Grilled Chicken

Serves 4

Marinade

1-1/2 cups macadamia nut oil

2/3 cups red wine vinegar

1 clove garlic, minced

1/2 teaspoon chopped fresh thyme

1 teaspoon fresh chopped rosemary leaves

1/3 cup grated parmesan cheese

1-1/2 teaspoon salt

1 teaspoon fresh ground pepper

4 roasted chicken breasts—skin on, with ribs

Tomato Bread

3 juicy, vine-ripened tomatoes, cut into 1-inch pieces

Salt and pepper

3 hick slices of good quality sourdough bread, cut into 1-inch cubes and toasted

1/2 red onion, chopped into a fine dice

Directions

In a mixing bowl, stir the marinade ingredients together well. Pour half the marinade over the chicken. Let it marinade at least 1/2 hour, turning once. While the chicken is marinating, prepare the tomato bread salad. Lightly season the tomato with salt and pepper. Mix the tomato, bread, and onion in a bowl. Pour the remaining marinade over this mixture, and season to taste. Allow to marinate. Grill the chicken over medium heat, turning occasionally for 25–30 minutes or until firm to the touch or juices run clear. To serve, divide the tomato salad evenly among four plates, and place the chicken on top.

Chapter 29

SAVORY SIDES

Double Baked Sweet Potato with Cheddar and Bacon

2 servings

Ingredients

1 small to medium-sized sweet potato

2 pieces bacon, cooked and crumbled

2 tablespoons butter

2 ounces cheddar cheese, shredded

kosher salt

fresh crushed black pepper

Directions

Cover the sweet potato with aluminum foil. Pierce the potato and the foil in several different locations, and bake in 425 degree F oven for 60 minutes or until tender. Remove and slice the potato in half lengthwise. Remove the insides of the potato, and place in a small bowl. Add the butter, cheese, and bacon, and mash together well. Season to taste, and spoon it back into the potato shell. Put back in the oven for 15 minutes or until the tops are browned.

Mac and Cheese to the Max

Serves 8

Ingredients

1 box (13.25 oz. or about 3.5 cups)
whole grain macaroni

4 cups shredded cheese (Use any combination of cheeses that you like.
For example: grated cheddar, grated Gruyere, and Brie diced into
cubes without the rind.)

1 whole egg and 2 egg whites, beaten

1-1/2 cups whole milk

1 dash of cayenne pepper

2 teaspoons prepared mustard

Salt

Black Pepper, freshly ground

1/4 cup Parmesan cheese

paprika

Directions

Preheat oven to 375 degrees F. Bring a large pot of salted water to a boil.
When water boils, add the dry pasta, stir and bring back to a boil, then
reduce heat and time for 9-10 minutes. (The pasta will cook more in the
oven, so be sure to stop cooking when it's still fairly al dente.) Pour pasta
into a colander placed in the sink to drain. Mix together the prepared
mustard, salt, pepper, eggs, and milk and whip together with a fork.
Put the drained pasta back into the pan you cooked it in, then pour the
milk mixture over pasta and mix. Add the cheese and stir. Spray a 9" by
12" glass casserole dish with macadamia nut oil, then pour the macaroni
mixture in and evenly distribute in the dish. Sprinkle Parmesan cheese
and paprika on top if desired. Bake uncovered for 30-35 minutes, or
until all cheese is melted and cheese on top is starting to brown slightly.

Mediterranean Couscous Salad

8 servings

Ingredients

3/4 cup vegetable broth

1 cup uncooked couscous

4 tablespoons macadamia nut oil

1 (14-ounce) can artichoke hearts, drained and coarsely chopped

10 ounces green chilies, finely diced

1/2 cup crumbled feta

1/4 cup pine nuts, toasted

1/4 cup pitted kalamata olives

2 green onions, chopped

1 garlic clove, minced

2 tablespoons chopped fresh basil

2 tablespoons chopped fresh mint

2 tablespoons chopped fresh parsley

Directions

Bring the broth to a boil in a heavy saucepan, then stir in the couscous. Cover, return to a boil and remove from heat. Let stand for 5 minutes. Drizzle in the oil, fluff with a fork, and let cool. Combine the couscous, the artichokes, and the next nine ingredients, tossing gently, serve.

Sweet Potato Gratin

Serves 8

Ingredients

1 pint heavy whipping cream

4 sprigs fresh thyme

2 bay leaves

15 black peppercorns

15 cloves garlic, smashed

unsalted butter for baking dish

4 medium sweet potatoes, cut into 1/8 inch slices using a mandolin

Salt

Black pepper, fresh ground

Directions

Place the cream in a saucepan over high heat. Add the thyme, bay leaves, peppercorns, and 12 cloves of garlic. Bring to a boil, and immediately lower to a simmer. Simmer for 15 to 20 minutes, until the cream takes on all the flavors. In the final few minutes of the cooking process, add the remaining 3 cloves of garlic. Strain and clean, and discard the solids.

Lightly butter a 12-inch round baking dish, and cover the surface with a layer of potato slices. Dust with salt and pepper, and spoon some of the cream mixture over the top. Repeat with another layer of potatoes, seasoning, and cream until the gratin reaches a height of 2 inches. Press down gently on the potatoes to bring the cream to the top. Cover with aluminum foil, and continue to cook until the top is browned or the gratin is done (when a knife slips easily into the center).

Chapter 30

Sweet and Sinful Desserts

Shh! We won't tell if you don't.

Macadamia Nut Crumb Crust

Makes 1 9-inch pie crust

Ingredients

1 cup macadamia nuts
(or, alternatively, almonds), toasted
1/2 cup miller's bran
1/4 cup Stevia
6 tablespoons macadamia nut oil

Directions

Preheat the oven to 350 degrees F. Put the nuts on a cookie sheet and toast for about 5 minutes or until just brown—do not overcook. Put the nuts, bran, Stevia, and oil into a food processor. Pulse until everything is crumbled together. Press this mixture into the bottom of a 9-inch pie pan and bake it for 10—12 minutes until lightly browned. Remove it from the oven, add your pie filings, according to the pie recipe's instructions. Or you can pre-bake a lot of these crusts, allow them to cool completely, and freeze them.

Crunchy Pears w/Chocolate Whipped Cream

1 serving

Ingredients

1 ripe pear

2 tablespoons peanut butter, natural, sugar-free

2 tablespoons granola, sugar-free

Chocolate Whipped Cream for garnish (optional)
  (see recipe below)

Directions

Wash and dry the pear. Cut it in half lengthwise and remove the seeds. Place the pear halves in a sundae dish and spread the nut butter into the cored area of the fruit and around the edges. Sprinkle granola on top. To make it extra special, top with Chocolate Whipped Cream.

Chocolate Whipped Cream

Makes 1 Cup

Ingredients

1 cup heavy cream

1 teaspoon lo-han, or Stevia to taste

1 tablespoon unsweetened cocoa

Directions

Pour the cream into a cold stainless steel bowl—I put mine in the freezer for up to one hour before using it—and, with an electric mixer, set on the highest speed, whip the cream until just before it starts to from peaks. Add the sweetener, if you would like, at this point continue to whip the cream. Add the unsweetened cocoa and whip until stiff peaks form.

Too-Good-To-Be-True Peanut Butter Cookies

12 servings: Serving size = 2 cookies

Ingredients

    1 cup almond flour

    1-1/2 teaspoons baking powder (nonaluminum kind)

    2 teaspoons vanilla extract

    1/2 cup water

    1/4 teaspoon liquid Stevia

    2 teaspoons butter, melted

    4 tablespoons all-natural, sugar-free, crunchy peanut butter (room temperature)

Directions

Preheat oven to 350 degrees. Combine the flour, baking powder, vanilla extract, water, and sweetener and mix vigorously, either by hand or with an electric mixer. Then add the melted butter and the peanut butter. Combine all the ingredients well until a batter is formed. Drop the batter in teaspoon-size lumps onto a greased cookie sheet and place in the oven for 12 to 15 minutes. Allow to cool before eating—if you can resist!

Coconut Cream Pie

4 servings

Ingredients

- 1 pound queso blanco, divided into 4 even pieces
- 8 ounces shredded, unsweetened coconut
- 8 ounces heavy cream
- 4 tablespoons sour cream
- 4 macadamia nuts

Directions

Put each slice of queso blanco onto an oven-ready dessert plate. Sprinkle with coconut, and place in a pre-heated 400 degree F oven for about 5 minutes or until the cheese starts to melt. Remove from heat, and allow to cool for 5 minutes. Pour the cream over each one; dollop with the sour cream and place one nut on top of each dollop of sour cream.

Ridiculously Delicious Raspberry Cheesecake Squares

8 servings

Ingredients

- 1 package sugar-free raspberry gelatin
- 1 cup boiling water
- 2 (8-ounce) packages cream cheese, softened

Directions

Sprinkle the gelatin into the boiling water, and stir until well dissolved. In a bowl, beat the cream cheese until it is very creamy. With the mixer running, add the gelatin, 1/4 cup at a time, and mix until thoroughly combined. Pour into an 8x8-inch pan and refrigerate until firm, about 2 hours.

Frozen Chocolate Mud Pie

10 servings

Ingredients

3/4 cup heavy cream

1/2 Cup crème fraiche

4 ounces unsweetened chocolate, chopped in a food processor

1/2 cup Xylitol

Chocolate Whipped Cream (see recipe on page 301)

1 Macadamia Nut Crumb Crust (see recipe on page 300)

Directions

Place all the ingredients into the top of a double boiler over hot water. Whisk until well blended and the mixture begins to form small bubbles along the outside rim. Remove the mixture from the heat, and continue whisking until the chocolate becomes shiny and begins to cool. Set it aside to cool, and make the topping. Spoon the cooled filling into a prebake shell. Top with Chocolate Whipped Cream. Serve immediately or refrigerate.

Tantalizing Chocolate Truffles

Ingredients

1/2 cup dried apricots

1/4 cup walnuts, chopped

1/4 cup dried figs

1/4 cup lemon juice, freshly squeezed

1/4 cup almonds, sliced

4 ounces unsweetened chocolate

Directions

Put the fruit and nuts into a food processor and chop until they're small. Add the lemon juice and chop again. Scrape the mixture into a bowl and taste it to see if more lemon juice is needed. Melt the chocolate in a heatproof bowl in the microwave for about 2 minutes or, preferably, over a double boiler, until it's just melted. Roll the fruit mixture into small balls. Using two forks, roll each ball in the melted chocolate. Place the balls on oiled foil to cool and set. If the chocolate gets too hard to work with, briefly reheat it.

Georgia Cheesecake

Serves 8

Crust

3/4 cup finely crushed pecans

1/2 cup oat or almond flour

1/2 teaspoon cinnamon

2-3 tablespoons Stevia (to suit your taste)

1/2 cup melted butter

Filling

3 (8-ounce) packages of cream cheese
or Neufchatel cheese softened

1 cup granulated Stevia

1 teaspoon vanilla

3 eggs

1/4 cup cream

1 small peach, sliced thin

Directions

Melt the butter in a microwave safe bowl. Add the crushed pecans, almond or oat flour, Stevia and cinnamon, stir to combine. Prepare a 9" spring-form pan with non-stick spray then spread the crust evenly on the bottom and 1" up the sides of the pan.

Bake at 375 degrees F for 10 minutes. For the filling, beat the cream cheese, Stevia and vanilla until smooth and creamy. Add the eggs and cream, beat until combined. Pour the filling into the prepared crust, being careful to fill only to the top of the crust, and bake for 45 minutes or until it appears set when shaken. Loosen the cake from the sides of the pan with a knife or spatula and allow to cool for 30 minutes. Remove the sides of the spring-form pan and cool completely. Chill in the refrigerator for 3-4 hours before serving. Top with a few fresh slices of peaches and serve.

Coconut Macadamiaroons

Yields: 16 servings

Ingredients:

8 ounces unsweetened shredded coconut

8 ounces almond flour (any nut flour can be used)

4 tablespoons macadamia nut oil

1 tablespoon sugar substitute

Directions

Combine all ingredients in a stainless steel bowl until well mixed. For each cookie, spoon a tablespoonful of the mixture onto a cookie sheet. Bake in a preheated 325-degree F oven for about 6 mintues or until the cookies just start to get browned. Remove from heat, and allow to cool on wire rack.

Sources

Part I: Simple Natural Secrets to Life's Annoying Ailments: The ultimate guide to everyday illness—from IBS to LDL

http://lyprinol.ro/studii/A%20History%20 of%20Lyprinol.pdf

Belkowski and Lawson, The Effect of Perna on Collagen-Induced Arthritis in Rats. Clemson University.

Ibid

"Towards the minimal amount of exercise for improving metabolic health: beneficial effects of reduced-exertion high-intensity interval training." *Eur J Appl Physiol.* 2012; 112(7): 2,767-2,775

"Claudin-14 regulates renal Ca++ transport in response to CaSR signalling via a novel microRNA pathway," *The EMBO Journal* 2012; 31: 1,999-2,012

"Vitamin D Inhibits Monocyte/Macrophage Proinflammatory Cytokine Production by Targeting MAPK Phosphatase-1." *The Journal of Immunology*; 188(5): 2,127-2,135

Vitamin D status and pain: analysis from the Health Survey for England among English adults aged 65 years and over ." *British Journal of Nutrition* 2012; 107(7): 1,080-1,084

"Bromelain treatment decreases neutrophil migration to sites of inflammation." *Clin Immunol* 2008; 128(1): 66-74

"The anti-inflammatory effects of methylsulfonylmethane on lipopolysaccharide-induced inflammatory responses in murine macrophages." *Biol Pharm Bull* 2009; 32(4): 651-656

"Mediterranean Diet Supplemented With Coenzyme Q10 Modifies the Expression of Proinflammatory and Endoplasmic Reticulum Stress–Related Genes in Elderly Men and Women," *The Journals of Gerontology: Series A*; 67A(1): 3-10

"Choosing between NSAID and arnica for topical treatment of hand osteoarthritis in a randomised, double-blind study." *Rheumatol Int* 2007; 27(6): 585-591

"Efficacy and safety of Curcuma domestica extracts in patients with knee osteoarthritis." *J Altern Complement Med* 2009; 15(8): 891-897

"Capsaicin and pain mechanisms," *British Journal of Anaethesia* 1995; 75:157-168

"Decreased slow wave sleep increases risk of developing hypertension in elderly men." *Hypertension* 2011; 58(4): 596-603

"The effectiveness of dried cranberries (Vaccinium macrocarpon) in men with lower urinary tract symptoms." *Br J Nutr* 2010; 104(8): 1,181-1,189

"Genetic research clarifies link between hypertension and vitamin D," ScienceDaily (www.sciencedaily. com), 6/10/13

"The Impact of Fish and Shellfish Consumption on Age-Related Macular Degeneration."*Ophthalmology.* 2010 Dec;117(12):2395-401.

"Prospective study of dietary fat and the risk of age-related macular degeneration." Am J Clin Nutr. February 2001 vol. 73 no. 2 209-218.

"Dietary carotenoids, vitamins A, C, and E, and advanced age-related macular degeneration. Eye disease case-control study group." JAMA. 1994 Nov 9;272(18):1413-20.

"A prospective, randomized double-blind, placebo-controlled study of safety and efficacy of a high-concentration full-spectrum extract of Ashwagandha root in reducing stress and anxiety in adults." Indian J Psychol Med. 2012 Jul;34(3):255-62

"Scientific basis for the therapeutic use of Withania somnifera (ashwagandha): a review." Altern Med Rev. 2000 Aug;5(4):334-46.

"Fruit, Mediterranean-style, and high-fat and -sugar diets are associated with the risk of night sweats and hot flushes in midlife: results from a prospective cohort study." Am J Clin Nutr. 2013 May;97(5):1092-9.

Kostoglou-Athanassiou I. "Therapeutic Applications of Melatonin." Ther Adv in Endo and Metab. 2013;4(1):13-24.

Lissoni P, et al. "A phase II study of tamoxifen plus melatonin in metastatic solid tumour patients." *Br J Cancer.* 1996 Nov;74(9):1466-8.

Lissoni P, et al. "Five years survival in metastatic non-small cell lung cancer patients treated with chemotherapy alone or chemotherapy and melatonin: a randomized trial. *J Pineal Res.* 2003 Aug;35(1):12-5.

Lissoni P, et al. "A randomized study with the pineal hormone melatonin versus supportive care alone in patients with brain metastases due to solid neoplasms." Cancer. 1994 Feb 1;73(3):699-701.

"Melatonin secretion and the incidence of type 2 diabetes." *JAMA.* 2013 Apr 3;309(13):1388-96.

American Academy of Neurology (AAN) 65th Annual Meeting. Abstract S40.005. Presented March 20, 2012.

Pilot investigation of the circadian plasma melatonin rhythm across the menstrual cycle in a small group of women with premenstrual dysphoric disorder. *PLoS One.* 2012;7(12):e51929.

Sprake EF, et al. "Vitamin D3 as a novel treatment for irritable bowel syndrome: single case leads to critical analysis of patient-centred data." *BMJ Case Rep.* 2012 Dec 13;2012.

Teixeira TF, et al. Potential mechanisms for the emerging link between obesity and increased intestinal permeability. *Nutr Res.* 2012 Sep;32(9):637-47.

"Prolonged fasting reduces IGF-1/PKA to promote hematopoietic-stem-cell-based regeneration and reverse immunosuppression."*Cell Stem Cell.* 2014 Jun 5;14(6):810-23

Singer F, et al. [Drug therapy of activated arthrosis. On the effectiveness of an enzyme mixture versus diclofenac]. *Wien Med Wochenschr.* 1996;146(3):55-8

Klein G, et al. [Reducing pain by oral enzyme therapy in rheumatic diseases]. *Wien Med Wochenschr.* 1999;149(21-22):577-80

Akhtar NM, et al. Oral enzyme combination versus diclofenac in the treatment of osteoarthritis of the knee–a double-blind prospective randomized study. *Clin Rheumatol.* 2004 Oct;23(5):410-5

Klein G, et al. Efficacy and tolerance of an oral enzyme combination in painful osteoarthritis of the hip. A double-blind, randomised study comparing oral enzymes with non-steroidal anti-inflammatory drugs. *Clin Exp Rheumatol.* 2006 Jan-Feb;24(1):25-30

J Clin Endocrinol Metab 2011; 96(4): 1,093-1,097

CMAJ 2010; 182(11): E526-E531

Diabetes 2002; 51(1): 7-18

Phytomedicine 2011;18(6):479-485

"Acute effects of Fraxinus excelsior L. seed extract on postprandial glycemia and insulin secretion on healthy volunteers." *J Ethnopharmacol* 2009; 126(2): 226-32

"Acute intake of mulberry leaf aqueous extract affects postprandial glucose response after maltose loading: Randomized double-blind placebo-controlled pilot study." *Journal of Functional Foods* 2013; 5(3): 1,502-1,506

J Med Food. 2007; 10(1): 41-48

Stanislavov R, et al. "Improvement of erectile function with Prelox: a randomized, double-blind, placebo-controlled, crossover trial." International Journal of Impotence Research. 2008: 20; 173–180

"The role of protein in weight loss and maintenance." Am J Clin Nutr. 2015 Apr 29. pii: ajcn084038.

"Defining meal requirements for protein to optimize metabolic roles of amino acids." Am J Clin Nutr 2015;101(Suppl):1330S–8S.

"New gluten-free ingredient may cause allergic reaction, expert warns." ScienceDaily.com, 8/25/14

"Defining Powerhouse Fruits and Vegetables: A Nutrient Density Approach." Prev Chronic Dis 2014; 11: 130390.

"Watercress supplementation in diet reduces lymphocyte DNA damage and alters blood antioxidant status in healthy adults." Am J Clin Nutr. 2007 Feb;85(2):504-10.

"In vivo modulation of 4E binding protein 1 (4E-BP1) phosphorylation by watercress: a pilot study." British Journal of Nutrition, 2010; 1.

"Phenethyl isothiocyanate inhibits oxidative phosphorylation to trigger reactive oxygen species-mediated death of human prostate

cancer cells." J Biol Chem. 2010 Aug 20;
285(34): 26558-69.

"Daily blueberry consumption improves
blood pressure and arterial stiffness in
postmenopausal women with pre- and stage
1-hypertension: a randomized, double-blind,
placebo-controlled clinical trial." J Acad Nutr
Diet. 2015 Mar; 115(3): 369-77

"Anthocyanins and phenolic acids from a wild
blueberry (Vaccinium angustifolium) powder
counteract lipid accumulation in THP-1-
derived macrophages." Eur J Nutr. 2015 Jan 17

Schaumberg DA, et al. "Relations of body fat
distribution and height with cataracts in men."
Am J Clin Nutr 2000; 72: 1495-502

J Ocul Pharmacol Ther. 2006 Feb; 22(1): 10-8

Babizhayev MA, et al. "Efficacy of
N-acetylcarnosine in the treatment of
cataracts." Drugs R D. 2002; 3(2): 87-103

"B-vitamin status and bone mineral density
and risk of lumbar osteoporosis in older
females in the United States." Am J Clin Nutr.
2015 Sep; 102(3): 687-94.

"Effects of folic acid supplementation on
hearing in older adults: a randomized,
controlled trial." Ann Intern Med 2007;
146(1): 1-9

"Serum immunoreactive-leptin concentrations
in normal-weight and obese humans." N Engl J
Med. 1996 Feb 1; 334(5): 292-5.

"Cross-sectional and longitudinal associations
between circulating leptin and knee cartilage
thickness in older adults." Ann Rheum Dis.
2015 Jan;74(1):82-8.

"Towards a pro-inflammatory and
immunomodulatory emerging role of leptin."
Rheumatology 2006;45:944–950.

"Evidence for a Key Role of Leptin in
Osteoarthritis." Arthritis & Rheumatism. 2003
Nov; 48(11): 3118–3129.

"Significance of Increased Leptin Expression in
Osteoarthritis Patients." PLoS One. 2015 Apr
20;10(4):e0123224.

"Correlation of synovial fluid leptin
concentrations with the severity of
osteoarthritis." Clin Rheumatol. 2009;
28:1431–1435.

"The evolving role of obesity in knee

osteoarthritis." Curr Opin Rheumatol. 2010
September; 22(5): 533–537.

"Do synovial leptin levels correlate with pain in
end stage arthritis?" International Orthopaedics
(SICOT) (2013) 37:2071–2079.

"Relationship between leptin and body mass and
metabolic syndrome in an adult population." Rev
Port Cardiol. 2012;31(11):711-719.

"Association of knee osteoarthritis with the
accumulation of metabolic risk factors such as
overweight, hypertension, dyslipidemia, and
impaired glucose tolerance in Japanese men
and women: the ROAD study." J Rheumatol.
2011 May;38(5):921-30.

"Metabolic syndrome and a course of
osteoarthrosis." Ter Arkh. 2007;79(10):13-20.

"Cross-sectional and longitudinal associations
between circulating leptin and knee cartilage
thickness in older adults." Ann Rheum Dis.
2015 Jan;74(1):82-8.

"The effects of an oral preparation containing
hyaluronic acid (Oralvisc®) on obese knee
osteoarthritis patients determined by pain,
function, bradykinin, leptin, inflammatory
cytokines, and heavy water analyses."
Rheumatol Int. 2015 Jan;35(1):43-52.

"Dark chocolate acutely improves walking
autonomy in patients with peripheral artery
disease." J Am Heart Assoc. 2014 Jul 2;3(4).
pii: e001072.

Ito T, et al. "Enzyme-treated asparagus extract
promotes expression of heat shock protein and
exerts anti-stress effects." J Food Sci. 2014 Mar;
79(3): H413-9. Epub 2014 Feb 5.

Waki H, et al. "Effect of Enzyme-treated
asparagus (ETAS™) on the Stress Response
Substance in a Clinical Trial." Presented at the
35th European Society for Clinical Nutrition
and Metabolism (ESPEN) Congress, Leipzig,
Germany. 2013.

Ogasawara J. "Inhibitory Effect of ETAS against
Amyloid Beta-induced Cellular Disorder in
PC12 Cells." Amino Up Chemical Co. Ltd.
Sapporo, Japan, no date.

Ito T, et al. "Effects of enzyme-treated
asparagus extract on heat shock protein 70,
stress indices, and sleep in healthy adult men."
J Nutr Sci Vitaminol (Tokyo). 2014; 60(4):

283-90

"The Prostate Health Index: a new test for the detection of prostate cancer." Ther Adv Urol. Apr 2014; 6(2): 74–77.

"Reduced Rate of Repeated Prostate Biopsies Observed in ConfirmMDx Clinical Utility Field Study." Am Health Drug Benefits. 2014 May; 7(3): 129-34.

"⊠-Tocopherol bioavailability is lower in adults with metabolic syndrome regardless of dairy fat co-ingestion: a randomized, double-blind, crossover trial." Am J Clin Nutr. 2015 Nov; 102(5): 1070-80.

"An Effect of Oak-Wood Extract (Robuvit®) on Energy State of Healthy Adults-A Pilot Study."

Phytother Res. 2015 Aug; 29(8): 1219-24.

"Robuvit® (Quercus robur extract) supplementation in subjects with chronic fatigue syndrome and increased oxidative stress. A pilot registry study." J Neurosurg Sci. 2015 Jun; 59(2): 105-17.

"Improved management of primary chronic fatigue syndrome with the supplement French oak wood extract (Robuvit®): a pilot, registry evaluation." Panminerva Med. 2014 Mar; 56(1): 63-72.

"French oak wood extract (Robuvit®) reduces the wheal and flare response to histamine and decreases capillary filtration in normal subjects." Minerva Biotecnol. 2013; 25(4): 199-205.

"Influence of oak wood polyphenols on cysteine, homocysteine and glutathione total levels and PON1 activities in human adult volunteers – a pilot study." Gen Physiol Biophys. 2015 Jan; 34(1): 73-80.

"Robuvit® (French oak wood extract) in the management of functional, temporary hepatic damage. A registry, pilot study." Minerva Med. 2014 Feb; 105(1): 41-50.

"French Oak Wood (Quercus robur) Extract (Robuvit) in Primary Lymphedema: A Supplement, Pilot, Registry Evaluation." Int J Angiol. 2015 Mar; 24(1): 47-54.

"Improvement of erectile function by a combination of French maritime pine bark and roburins with amino acids." Minerva Urol Nefrol 2015 Mar;67(1): 27-32.

"Sperm quality in men is improved by supplementation with a combination of L-arginine, L-citrullin, roburins and Pycnogenol®." Minerva Urol Nefrol 2014 Dec; 66(4):2 17-23

"Validating bifidobacterial species and subspecies identity in commercial probiotic products." Pediatr Res. 2015 Nov 16.

"Effects of ⊠-lipoic acid and eicosapentaenoic acid in overweight and obese women during weight loss." Obesity (Silver Spring). 2015 Feb; 23(2): 313-21.

"Rapid and accurate determination of malate, citrate, pyruvate and OAA by enzymatic reactions coupled to formation of a fluorochromophore: Application in colorful juices and fermentable food (yogurt, wine) analysis." Food Chemistry. 15 November 2011; 129(2): 608–613.

"Pyruvate dehydrogenase activity in osmotically shocked rat brain mitochondria: stimulation by OAA." J Neurochem. 1988 Mar; 50(3): 673-80.

"The stressed synapse: the impact of stress and glucocorticoids on glutamate transmission." Nature Reviews Neuroscience. 2012 Jan; 13: 22-37

"The Effect of Blood Glutamate Scavengers OAA and Pyruvate on Neurological Outcome in a Rat Model of Subarachnoid Hemorrhage." Neurotherapeutics. 2012 Jul; 9(3): 649–657.

"OAA supplementation increases lifespan in Caenorhabditis elegans through an AMPK/ FOXO-dependent pathway." Aging Cell. 2009 Dec; 8(6): 765–768

"High blood glutamate OAA transaminase levels are associated with good functional outcome in acute ischemic stroke." J Cereb Blood Flow Metab. 2011 Jun; 31(6): 1387-93.

"OAA activates brain mitochondrial biogenesis, enhances the insulin pathway, reduces inflammation and stimulates neurogenesis." Hum Mol Genet. 2014 Dec 15; 23(24): 6528-41.

"Glutamine Addiction: A New Therapeutic Target in Cancer." Trends Biochem Sci. 2010 Aug; 35(8): 427–433.

"Blood glutamate scavengers prolong the survival of rats and mice with brain-implanted gliomas." Invest New Drugs. 2012 Feb 2.

Part II: Shockingly Simple Cures for Today's Biggest Killers

"Impaired neurovascular repair in subjects with diabetes following experimental intracutaneous axotomy," *Brain* 2011; 134(6): 1,853-1,863

The JUPITER trial: results, controversies, and implications for prevention. Ridker PM. Center for Cardiovascular Disease Prevention, Division of Preventive Medicine, Brigham and Women's Hospital, Harvard Medical School, Boston, Mass 02215, USA. pridker@partners.org

Lyon Diet Heart Study: Benefits of a Mediterranean-Style, National Cholesterol Education Program/American Heart Association Step I Dietary Pattern on Cardiovascular Disease Penny Kris-Etherton, PhD, RD; Robert H. Eckel, MD; Barbara V. Howard, PhD; Sachiko St. Jeor, PhD, RD; Terry L. Bazzarre, PhD; for the Nutrition Committee, Population Science Committee, and Clinical Science Committee of the American Heart Association

SSC International Collaborative Study to establish the first high fibrinogen plasma reference material for use with different fibrinogen assay techniques N. WEINSTOCK, M. NTEFIDOU,THE ISTH/ SSC FIBRINOGEN SUBCOMMITTEE AND THE GTH FIBRINOGEN WORKING PARTY 25 MAY 2006

A prospective study of fibrinogen and risk of myocardial infarction in the physicians' health study Jing Ma, MD, PhD, Charles H Hennekens, MD, DrPH, Paul M Ridker, MD, Meir J *Stampfer*, Volume 33, Issue 5, April 1999, Pages 1347-1352

Plasma fibrinogen — a major coronary risk factor M.C. Stone and J.M. Thorp J R Coll Gen Pract. 1985 December; 35(281): 565–569.

Increased markers of thrombogenesis in chronic atrial fibrillation: effects of warfarin treatment Gregory Y H Lip, Gordon D 0 Lowe, Ann Rumley, Francis G Dunn Br HeartJf 1995;73:527-533

A prospective study of fibrinogen and risk of myocardial infarction in the physicians' health study, Jing Ma, MD, PhD, Charles H Hennekens, MD, DrPH, Paul M Ridker, MD, Meir J Stampfer, Volume 33, Issue 5, April 1999, Pages 1347–1352

Variable Hypocoagulant Effect of Fish Oil Intake in Humans Modulation of Fibrinogen Level and Thrombin Generation Kristof Vanschoonbeek, Marion A.H. Feijge, Martine Paquay, Jan Rosing, Wim Saris, Cornelis Kluft, Peter L.A. Giesen, Moniek P.M. de Maat, Johan W.M. Heemskerk Published online before print June 24, 2004

A Systemic Review of the Roles of n-3 Fatty Acids in Health and Disease NATALIE D. RIEDIGER, MSc*; RGIA A. OTHMAN, MSc*; MIYOUNG SUH, PhD, RD; MOHAMMED H. MOGHADASIAN, PhD

Male pattern baldness and its association with coronary heart disease: a meta-analysis," BMJ Open 2013; 3(4): pii: e002537

Heart disease and C-reactive protein (CRP) testing," WebMD (www.webmd.com), accessed 9/24/13

"Level of fibrinogen and risk of fatal and non-fatal stroke. EUROSTROKE: a collaborative study among research centres in Europe," J Epidemiol Community Health 2002; 56(Suppl I): i14-i18

"Undetectable high-sensitivity cardiac troponin T level in the emergency department and risk of myocardial infarction," *Journal of the American College of Cardiology* 2014; 63(23): 2,568-2,578

"Blood test shows promise for gauging heart attack risk after chest pain," *U.S. News and World Report* (www.health.usnews.com), 3/31/14

"Automated External Defibrillators can save lives during cardiac emergencies," Office of Safety and Health Administration (www.osha.gov), accessed 7/29.14

"Comparison of naïve sixth-grade children with trained professionals in the use of an Automated Esternal Defibrillator," *Circulation* 1999; 100: 1,703-1,707

"Preventing Alzheimer's disease-related gray matter atrophy by B-vitamin treatment," PNAS 2013; May 20 (epub ahead of print)

"Cognitive and clinical outcomes of homocysteine-lowering B-vitamin treatment in mild cognitive impairment: a randomized controlled trial." *Int J Geriatr Psychiatry*. 2012; 27(6): 592-600

"Four Clinical Trials Further Clarify The Role Of Physical Activity In Cognitive Function And Dementia," PRNewswire (www.prnewswire.

com), 7/15/12

"Predicting cognitive decline: A dementia risk score vs the Framingham vascular risk scores." *Neurology.* 2013;80(14):1300-6.

"Cognitive improvement in mild to moderate Alzheimer's dementia after treatment with the acetylcholine precursor choline alfoscerate: a multicenter, double-blind, randomized, placebo-controlled trial." *Clin Ther* 2003; 25(1): 178-193

"Choline alphoscerate in cognitive decline and in acute
 cerebrovascular disease: an analysis of published clinical data." *Mech Ageing Dev* 2001; 122(16): 2,041-2,055

"Influence of vascular comorbidities on the antioxidant
defense system in Alzheimer's disease," *Deutsche Medizinische Wochenschrift* 2012; 137(7): 305-8

"Nutritional intervention in brain aging: reducing the effects
of inflammation and oxidative stress," *Subcell Biochem*
2007; 42: 299-318

"Magnesium Modulates Amyloid-Protein Precursor
Trafficking and Processing," *Journal of Alzheimer's Disease* 2010; 20(4): 1,091-1,106

"Dietary Intakes of Vitamin E, Vitamin C, and Beta-Carotene, and Risk of Alzheimer's Disease: A Meta-Analysis," *Journal of Alzheimer's Disease* 2012; 31(2): 253-258

 "Nutritional determinants of cognitive aging and dementia," *Proceedings of the Nutrition Society* 2012; 71(1): 1-13

"Compartmental neck fat accumulation and its relation to cardiovascular risk and metabolic syndrome," *Am J Clin Nutr* 2014; 100(5): 1,244-1,251

Neck Circumference as an Independent Predictive Contributor to Cardio-Metabolic Syndrome," *Cardiovasc Diabetol.* 2013;12(76)

"Self-reported sleep disturbance is associated with Alzheimer's disease risk in men," *Alzheimer's & Dementia,* epub ahead of print 10/27/14

Mastroiacovo D, et al. "Cocoa flavanol consumption improves cognitive function, blood pressure control, and metabolic profile in elderly subjects: the Cocoa, Cognition, and Aging (CoCoA) Study—a randomized controlled trial." Am J Clin Nutr. February 2015 ajcn.092189; First published online December 17, 2014.

Brickman AM, et al. "Enhancing dentate gyrus function with dietary flavanols improves cognition in older adults." Nat Neurosci. 2014 Dec;17(12):1798-803. Epub 2014 Oct 26.

National Multiple Sclerosis Society. Vitamin D. http://www.nationalmssociety.org/Research/Research-News-Progress/Vitamin-D. Accessed March 3, 2015.

American Academy of Neurology. "People with Multiple Sclerosis May Have Lower Levels of Key Nutrients." https://www.aan.com/PressRoom/Home/PressRelease/1343. Accessed March 3, 2015.

"Investigation of a Melissa officinalis special extract on Cognition I: In vitro study on muscarinic properties." Agro Food Industry Hi Tech. Jan/Feb 2015; 26(1)

"Anti-Stress Effects of Lemon Balm-Containing Foods." Nutrients. 2014; 6: 4805-4821

"Investigation of a Melissa officinalis special extract on Cognition II: Human study – Lemon balm extract administered in confectionary bars." Agro Food Industry Hi-Tech, Mar/Apr 2015; 26(2): 12-14

Zhao, J. "Cancer stem cells and chemoresistance: The smartest survives the raid." Pharmacology & Therapeutics. 2016; 160: 145–158

Al-Hajj M, et al. "Prospective identification of tumorigenic breast cancer cells." Proc Natl Acad Sci USA. 2003 Apr 1; 100(7): 3983-8

Sordillo PP & Helson L. "Curcumin and cancer stem cells: curcumin has asymmetrical effects on cancer and normal stem cells." Anticancer Res. 2015 Feb; 35(2): 599-614

Lagadec C, et al. "Radiation-induced reprograming of breast cancer cells." Stem Cells 2012 May; 30(5): 833–844

He ZY, et al. "Upregulation of p53 Expression in Patients with Colorectal Cancer by Administration of Curcumin." Cancer Investigation. 2011; 29: 208–213

Gupta SC, et al. "Therapeutic Roles of Curcumin: Lessons Learned from Clinical Trials." AAPS J. 2013 Jan; 15(1): 195-218

Mimeault M. & Batra SK. "Potential applications of curcumin and its novel synthetic analogs and nanotechnology-based formulations in cancer prevention and therapy." Chinese Medicine. 2011, 6: 31

Kumar A, et al. "Curcumin Resource Database." Database. 2015, 1–6

Baharuddin P, et al. "Curcumin improves the efficacy of cisplatin by targeting cancer stem-like cells through p21 and cyclin D1-mediated tumour cell inhibition in non-small cell lung cancer cell lines." Oncol Rep. 2016 Jan; 35(1): 13–25. Published online 2015 Nov 2

Cheng AL, et al. "Phase I clinical trial of curcumin, a chemopreventive agent, in patients with high-risk or pre-malignant lesions." Anticancer Res. 2001; 21: 2895-2900

Cuomo J, et al. "Comparative Absorption of a Standardized Curcuminoid Mixture and Its Lecithin Formulation." J Nat Prod, 2011 Apr 25; 74(4): 664-9

Howells LM, et al. "Curcumin ameliorates oxaliplatin-induced chemoresistance in HCT116 colorectal cancer cells in vitro and in vivo." Int J Cancer. 2011 Jul 15; 129(2): 476-86

Chandra D, et al. "Cryoablation and Meriva have strong therapeutic effect on triple-negative breast cancer." Oncoimmunology. 2016; 5(1): e1049802. Published online 2015 May 29

Irving GR, et al. "Combining curcumin (C3-complex, Sabinsa) with standard care FOLFOX chemotherapy in patients with inoperable colorectal cancer (CUFOX): study protocol for a randomised control trial." Trials. 2015; 16: 110.

Sharma RA, et al. "Pharmacodynamic and Pharmacokinetic Study of Oral Curcuma Extract in Patients with Colorectal Cancer." Clin Cancer Res. 2001 Jul; 7(7): 1894-900

Bayet-Robert M, et al. "Phase I dose escalation trial of docetaxel plus curcumin in patients with advanced and metastatic breast cancer." 2010. Cancer Biology & Therapy. 9: 1, 8-14

Part III: The New Hamptons Health Miracle: The next generation cure for diabetes, pre-diabetes, belly fat, metabolic syndrome, and so much more

"How non-consumption shapes desire," *Journal of Consumer Research* 2014; 41(4): 936